The Heavenly Program

~Harmonizing with the Spiritual Influence in Nature~

Masaru Kawai

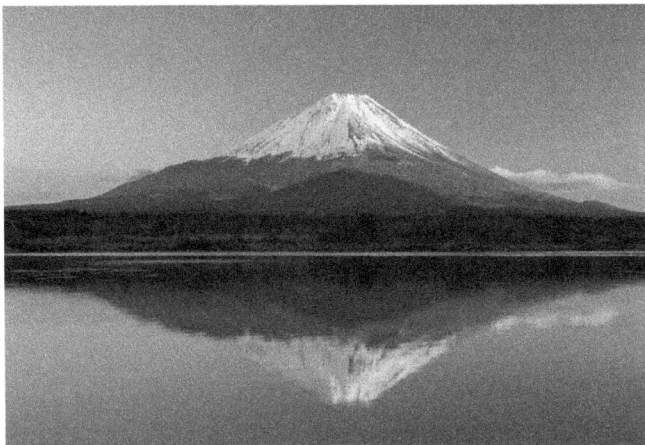

Copyright: shihina / 123RF Photos

Translator: Kanae Ervin
Proofreader: Arthur Coleman
Coordinator: Junko Rodriguez
Publisher: Miyoko Yuasa

Cover photo copyrighted © by Hiromi Suzuki

Published by Babel Press U.S.A.

ISBN: 978-0991478927

Babel Corporation
Pacific Business News Bldg. #208,
1833 Kalakaua Avenue, Honolulu, Hawaii 96815

Table of Contents

Foreword

The modern society is in a chaotic state.

Science cannot reverse the damages done to the nature on this planet. Most scientist are hopeless that the future cannot be predicted. Many diseases have not been fully researched as to how they develop, therefore the only treatments available are either to remove by operating or kill off the sickened cells.

The idea of God that humans and their religious beliefs hold were conceived through the dogma of humans, and has always been in conflict with others. In truth, God is the principle of the exchanges between atoms and electrons. This is the first book in the world that reveals this truth.

This book will also touch upon the Super Consciousness, which gives us the wisdoms of the domain of God almighty through telepathy. I will now give you some insights about these wisdoms.

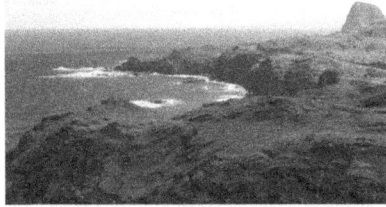

CHAPTER ONE

Right now, *throughout the world, destructive behavior is occurring toward the creation of a Utopian society. The rise of the Trump administration is also part of the heavenly world's program. This is a message to modern people from the heavenly world (God the Father, Moses, Jesus) --- What characterizes this new era?*

1. The world is currently in a state of chaos. Why? Because a program is being carried out by the heavenly world. Our world is moving along according to this program in order for the Utopian society to soon be realized.

This is the program of the heavenly world; everything that happens on this planet is ruled by invisible laws. Understanding the plans of the heavenly world and the rules governing everything, we can predict the future. Nothing that happens in this world on any given day is an accident. Natural disasters, abnormal weather events, accidents and other calamities all occur according to the invisible laws and other karmic rules. The heavenly world decides the history and the future of all human beings, societies, nations, and ethnic groups.

The Creator, whom Jesus called the Father, is the sole God who forged the universe, the natural world and the human world. The higher-dimensional consciousness that comes from the Father now moves in the consciousness of Moses and Jesus. The law of the universe is the law of love, harmony and circulation. It is the idea of 'give & give.'

Human society works on the basis of the idea of 'Give & take', but many people nowadays want to 'take & take.' The desire for more money, more material goods, and the idea that any behavior can be justified "as long as I'm okay" prevail. The world in this condition is in its latter days. It is a world in the Kali Yuga age. From now on, whoever does not carry out the law of love will be judged as unnecessary in society, and will be erased by accidents, mishaps or natural disasters. According to the program of the heavenly world, in a mere several years, the Earth will become a Utopian society. It will become one world, a world without borders in which all conflicts and wars will cease.

All religions, science and philosophy will be united under the law of the Universe, which is the absolute truth that abides forever. All conflicts will vanish.

In the heavenly world, the layout and blueprints for the Utopian society have already been completed. Those who are not included in this blueprint are obstructive or unnecessary for the realization of the Utopian society. They will be eliminated and disappear.

In order to realize and create the Utopian society, the destruction of evil is necessary. This destruction began in the 21st century and should be completed by the end of 2017. The Utopian society will be realized. Right now, destruction for the sake of creation is taking place. You are hereby introduced to the content of the heavenly world's program, including how the global economy and political environment will change, how the industries of the 21st century may begin to operate under the universally-governing law, and how to heal intractable diseases. The meaning of the birth of the newly established Trump administration lies here as well.

2. The time to understand the true meaning of "Oh my God!" -- is NOW.

Currently, the world is beset by conflict. Killings and other acts of violence are being carried out by terrorists because of conflicts between religions. The newly established Trump administration in the United States has divided public opinion within that nation. In other developed countries also, public opinion is in conflict, and is constantly swaying from one side to the other.

When something unexpected occurs, people will call upon God for salvation by saying, "Oh my God." The heavenly world, or the world of God, is the root cause of the creation of the Universe, the natural world and human society. Today, the heavenly world is forcing the mundane world into a quagmire.

People look up to the sky instead of looking down. They shout out, in their minds, "Oh my God! Isn't God there?" Such is the present state.

The only God, the Creator and Father in the heavenly world is the very one who created the Universe, the natural world and the human world. The Father told Moses, "I am that I am." Jesus's disciples asked him, "What is God?" To which he replied, "God is Almighty. God is Everything.

The Creator created the law that dominates everything. All 100% of things in this world are subject to this law. To God are attributed the eternal laws that govern even atoms and electrons (energy and material, according to Einstein). We humans, through our daily dramas, have conceived our own ideas of God. But the law of the Creator is absolutely consistent, and it dominates all events that happen on the Earth and in the Universe. Moreover, there is a system that assists whoever obeys this law, while it imposes judgement and carries out restitution to cleanse the sins of the lawbreakers and makers of negative karma. This system also works to diminish the effects karma.

For example, the heavenly world warns that the nuclear power is dangerous and should not be developed. The accidents that happened at the Three Mile Island, Chernobyl and Fukushima nuclear power plants were all caused by the heavenly world as a means of sending a warning to humanity. Stop developing such dangerous technology. Have the wisdom to cope when an accident occurs.

However, humans are not reflecting on such accidents, and they continue to generate nuclear power. Ignoring this warning, the heavenly world cautions, will lead to an even bigger accident. At the G7 Summit held in Japan in 2016, former US President Obama offered paper cranes at the atomic bomb dome memorial in Hiroshima. However, the US government did not issue an official apology to the atomic bomb victims.

The heavenly world, through Mr. Yoshihide Uezu who was dispatched to Japan in the 20th century as a Japanese person, is sending a warning in an attempt to guide humanity; "If Americans do not apologize to the victims of the nuclear weapons dropped on Hiroshima and Nagasaki, there will be a nuclear disaster within the United States that will far worse than those in Hiroshima and Nagasaki," it warns.

The council of the highest level of the heavenly world that is guiding humanity is called Shambhala. The Utopian society is known as Shangri-la.

There are seven entrances on this Earth that lead to the world of Shambhala. Its headquarters is under Mt. Lhotse in the Himalayas. The headquarters of the entire galaxy is located in the Pleiades constellation. (See the photo on the next page).

There are 33 members of the Shambhala council in the 21st century - three with physical bodies, and the rest being higher-dimensional consciousness entities such as Moses, Buddha, and Jesus Christ. The council is chaired by the Creator.

The leader of the three human members is Mr. Toshihiko Chibana, a Japanese citizen. I, the author, spent 17 years working alongside Mr. Chibana, and was able to obtain information from him about the heavenly world. I will now reveal the contents of this information in my report.

Most of the venues for this council are located within Toyama Prefecture, which has the highest energy frequencies in Japan. In the

The Seven Chakras of the World

Seventh Chakra

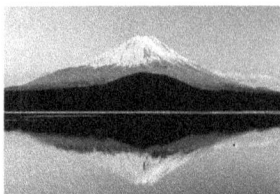

Copyright: shihina / 123RF Photos

Mt. Fuji in Japan

Fifth Chakra

Sixth Chakra

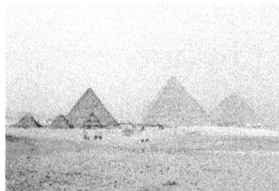

Great Pyramid of Giza

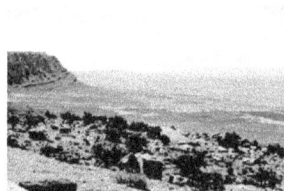

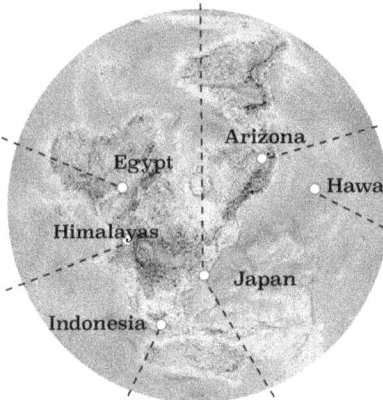

Navajo and Hopi reservation

Arizona

Egypt

Hawaii

Himalayas

Fourth Chakra

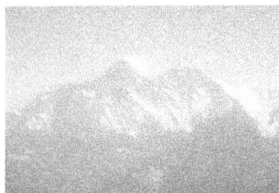

First Chakra

Japan

Indonesia

Himalayas

The view of the world from the North Pole

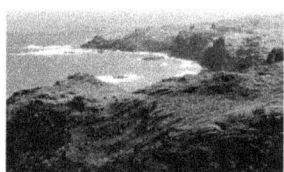

Copyright: ChristopherKelleher / 123RF Photos

Maui, Hawaii

Second Chakra

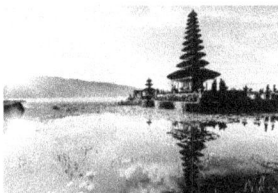

Third Chakra

Copyright: GalynaAndrushko / 123RF Photos

Bali, Indonesia

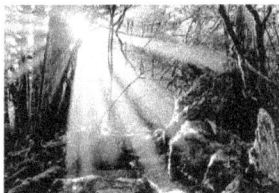

Copyright: Hiromi Suzuki

Yakushima, Japan

1. Tail bone | The entrance of the basic energy | Maui, Hawaii – holds the strongest residual power of Mu civilization
2. Abdomen | The fundamental energy for all human activities | Bali, Indonesia
3. Stomach | Energy for ideas and spirit | Yakushima, Japan – the 'bellybutton' of the world, home of ancient Jomon Cedar trees
4. Heart | The most important spot of the body, the center | Himalayas – emits the pure white energy
5. Throat | Creations and wisdom | Great Pyramid – the energy spot for creation and wisdom
6. Forehead | Foresight, insight | Navajo and Hopi reservations – the very accurate Hopi prophecies
7. Crown | Interactions and unification with God | Mt. Fuji, Japan – the final destination of all humankind

underground levels of the Shambhala headquarters in the Himalayas, as of right now, there are 7.6 billion lamps lit. This equates to the number of people who now live on Earth as human beings. When a person's consciousness is high, the light is brighter; when low, it is dimmer. The Guiding Spirit watches over the state of each person, enabling the heavenly world to guide whoever has the brightest light.

The Shambhala council dictates the evolution of mankind. Their objects of focus include all individuals, groups, nations, ethnic groups, and so on. They carry out the planning, timing and implementation of all kinds of natural disasters, abnormal weather events, accidents, calamities, etc., as well as all positive world events that occur.

There is a distinction between natural disasters and human disasters. Human disasters occur when people break the Law, and since the responsibility for these disasters rests on the person who broke the Law, this person who transgresses the law should be eliminated. They end up liquidating their sins. There are reasons people die in earthquakes, natural disasters or accidents, man-made or otherwise. We must all understand that it is the council that controls them.

3. The heavenly world sends the Earth the leaders of the human race as needed.

The leaders are sent to the Earth whenever necessary, in order to realize the evolution of humanity. Some of the most significant leaders are listed chronologically.

Moses was dispatched some 3,200 years ago. He was bestowed the Ten Commandments and gave us the Old Testament.

Buddha was dispatched approximately 2,500 years ago to preach the Law and compassion. He gave us Buddhism.

Jesus was dispatched about 2,000 years ago. He preached love, and gave us the New Testament.

Today, four Japaneses and 12 others, including Indians and Americans, have been dispatched on the Earth.

In 1991, Mr. Toshihiko Chibana, the leader of the human constituent of the heavenly council, along with Mr. Yoshikichi Sukeyasu, both Japanese citizens, have received messages from Moses, Buddha and Jesus Christ to give to modern people.

Message from Moses (from "The New Ten Commandment and the Newer Ten Commandments" by Yoshikichi Sukeyasu, published by the Eight Company)

①Today, our 3,200-year history is about to be re-written. Humanity's consciousness had declined in the past 3,200 years. Material civilization has developed, but spiritual civilization has degenerated. For this reason, it has become a lawless era. This period is called the latter days. What have the last 3,200 years of history been for? Earthlings, you must wake up right now!

②If a person retains even an iota of selfishness, desire or an inability to understand the invisible dimensions, a storm of purification will blow through the Earth, ending the period of training for that person's physical body; at this point, the training period in the spiritual world begins. No one will be able to go against this movement. No matter how hard people may resist, the foundation will collapse and crumble.

③This shift to a new era has already begun in 1989. The transformation from the old values and materialistic desires for reputation, status, money and power to new values that transcend life and death and hold across race, religion, economy, science and all areas - will lead us to a mindfulness-centered lifestyle. The new era will have no physical-bodied leader. Whoever cannot adapt to the changes of this era will be raised to the spiritual dimension immediately. That is, a storm of purification will blow through the Earth and end all the training period of people in their physical bodies.

The requirements for leaders in this new era are: ① Have no selfishness, ② Be able to take immediate actions, ③ Leave everything to the higher-dimensional spirits and be open for them to work through you. Currently there is hardly anybody who fulfills all of these requirements. This is why the evolution of mankind has been delayed.

Message from the Buddha, given through Yoshikichi Sukeyasu via his book, "The Way to Hope" published by the Eight Company.

◦None of the events and phenomena on this Earth occur by chance. They all happen according to the work of the heavenly consciousness. Things happen according to the laws of cause and effect. Having greed and obsession will result in an instant loss of energy. This world is indeed in its latter days.

Message from Jesus, given in 1991, through Yoshikichi Sukeyasu via his book, "The New Sermon on the Mount" published by the Eight Company.
◦The upcoming new era will be an era of great harmony. There will

be no war, trouble among races, nor conflict among religions nor among nations. In the new era, everything will be one. All nations, religions, science and human beings will be joined together as one to enter the era of harmony on Earth.

4. The latest message from the heavenly world (given by the Creator, Moses, Jesus Christ and other higher-dimensional conscious entities through Mr. Yoshihide Uezu and Mr. Toshihiko Chibana)

* Mr. Uezu was dispatched in the 20th century, along with Mr. Chibana and Mr. Uezu, for the guidance of humanity.

(1) The program of human evolution is in motion. In 2012, the Earth entered a dimension of higher energy. The energy has been becoming stronger year by year. The purpose of this program is for humanity to evolve from the 'emotional type' to the 'rational type,' then ultimately to the 'spiritual type.' People of the emotional type have lower energy and coarse vibrations. They insist on obtaining money and material goods, and their attitude comes down to 'me-first.' The rational type of people, on the other hand, can control their emotions with their mental energy. They propagate the 'give and give' attitude. They practice coexistence and co-prosperity, helping and sharing with each other. This process is sometimes called the photon belt or ascension. The emotional type of people tend to cause fights and conflicts, are mentally stressed out, and emit destructive vibrations which end up pooling in underground plates and causing natural disasters, abnormal weather events, accidents and other calamities.

People of this type are those who are not needed in the realization of the Utopian society of the heavenly world, therefore they will be eliminated.

(2) Today, time on Earth is becoming relatively faster. There used to be time for reflection when someone broke a law, but no such time remains now. Disasters or accidents will come to him or her immediately. The path of one's life used to be relatively smooth. But nowadays, it is rather like a steep slope or a cliff. Those whose mind is clouded will not be able to climb the cliff, and will be eliminated.

(3) The absolute truths and the eternal laws of the universe.

① −　　—　　+　　The law of Yin and Yang
②　　　　|　　　　The law of cause and effect
③ −　◯◯　+　The law of energy circulation.

These three laws control all phenomena at 100% recall rate. In the very near future, every religion, science and philosophy will be absorbed entirely. Conflicts will disappear. The combination of the symbols [−] and [|] form the law of the 'cross' [+].

The materialistic civilization will collapse and be replaced by a spiritual civilization. The collapse of the bubble will occur without fail. No human being will ever be able to take their share away with them. The economies of developed countries are already imploding. The collapse of the economy will lead to the collapse of the political system. Within four to five years from now, all borders of the world will disappear. The world will be as one, and all wars will cease. At this point, the world leader will be a Japanese national. This scenario is according to the program of the heavenly world. The construction of a new system that will lead to the realization of the Utopian society will begin in the year 2020.

Today, throughout the world, we witness paranormal phenomena, abnormal movements in the economic and political world, natural disasters, abnormal weather events, accidents and other calamities. None of these happen by chance. Their occurrence is inevitable. They are caused by the state of people's minds, especially those who stir up karma by breaking the law of the universe. The elimination process comes about as those phenomena. This is what we call the Last Judgment, or Armageddon.

President Trump has approved exploratory boring for the production of shale oil and the construction of pipelines that will contaminate the natural environment. Furthermore, he is rejuvenating the coal industry. The CO_2 emissions from coal will destroy the environment further and accelerate global warming.

He proposed the US' withdrawal from the international agreement for environmental protection. Global warming will accelerate steadily. Russia's Arctic permafrost will melt, releasing deadly viruses and dinosaur bones. (Today in the Arctic, potato flowers bloom in parts of the permafrost. The destruction of the natural environment, coupled with the fact that we now try to kill microorganisms that are considered harmful germs, is starting to trigger a counterattack on the part of these microorganisms against the mankind. There are more outbreaks by devastating viral diseases. Modern medicine is not equipped to handle them. A large number of these occurrences are seen in the desert regions of the world and in China. The destructive vibrations that come from people desiring more money and material goods and have self-centered attitudes are generating new types of devastating viruses.

The Utopian society will soon be realized. For that to happen, it is necessary to destroy the people and the systems that emit such destructive vibrations. The process of destruction that must take place in order for creation to happen started at the beginning of the 21st century, and will soon be at its peak. The Earth will become a sacred planet in the near future.

The program of the heavenly world is to hand over the leadership of the world to Japanese people in the 21st century. The Earth is a rotating sphere, a flowing ball. Okinawa used to be called Ryukyu (meaning 'flowing ball'). Starting in 2017, Okinawa will be the center of the civilization of the minds.

The Shambhala conferences are held in Japan. Both Moses as far back as 3,200 years ago and Jesus, 2,000 years ago, used to be members of this council as physical-bodied humans. Both of them used to join the conferences held in Japan with their consciousness by leaving their physical bodies, then returning to them afterwards. They talked with many Japanese people in various parts of Japan.

There are many sacred spots in different parts of Japan where Moses and Jesus supposedly talked to people in those days.

In Japan, the tomb of Moses is in Mt. Hodatsu, Noto Peninsula. The tomb of Jesus is located in Herai village in Aomori prefecture. According to the locals, the name "Herai" derived from "Hebrew."

The Japanese people and the Jewish people are connected like two sides of a coin. "Kojiki (A Record of Ancient Matters)," a book published in the year 720 in Japan, notes that Jewish people, who represent the rational type in the new era, will support the Japanese people in the 21st century.

In the latter chapters in this book, the specific contents of the law of the universe will be introduced.

5. The phenomena occurring in the world today indicate the collapse of the system of the old era, which is the materialistic civilization.

Major cataclysmic changes in politics and the economy are occurring in developed countries.

No one could have accurately predicted the remarkable changes that have happened in the world. They were unexpected, and history will repeat itself.

○ 1989 Collapse of the Berlin Wall and Tiananmen Incident in China.

○ 1990 Collapse of the dictatorships in Romania and Mongolia.

○ 1991 Collapse of the Soviet Union and communism. The first burst of the economic bubble in the world occurred in Japan (about 10 trillion USD lost).

○ 2016 Brexit in the UK. The rise of the Trump administration.

○ 2016 - 2017 Frequent abnormal phenomena throughout the world. Reference: Earth Catastrophe Review (Japanese website, www. http://earthreview.net/)

Acceleration of global warming. Arctic permafrost defrosts and potato flowers bloom. Heavy snowfall in Africa. Death of fish en masse. The most frequent number of volcanic eruptions in recorded history. The most frequent number of large-scale earthquakes in recorded history.

○ **Economic phenomena**

•Loans at negative interest rates continue: Currently valued at 1,000 trillion yen (89 trillion dollars) worldwide. There are no good investment destinations for funds.

•US national debt: 2,200 trillion yen (195 trillion $) --- There is no way of repaying this.

- China's national debt: 3,300 trillion yen (292 trillion $) --- There is no way of repaying this.
- EU banks: Increase in nonperforming loans due to the decline of real estate valuations. Economic crisis.
- Estimated 340 trillion yen (3 trillion dollars) in local government's debt to China: 4 times Japan's national budget.
- China's outstanding loans by shadow banks: 680 trillion yen (6 trillion $)

Non-performing loans in China: Approximately 500 trillion yen (4.4 trillion $).

Illegal accumulation of wealth by Chinese bureaucrats: 250 trillion yen (1.1 trillion $). Most of these funds went overseas.

Because people do not believe in the future of their own countries:

- 60 million refugees worldwide, 24 million refugees leaving their own countries.

○ **Phenomena occurring in the world**

- Globalization has resulted in winner-takes-all situations in the developing economies that offer cheaper-cost goods. It has also resulted in the decline of the manufacturing industry in developed countries, lower income for people and fewer opportunities for higher education, the spreading of grudges, and suffering and hatred being the predominant emotions in "my country first" ways of thinking.
- The quantitative expansion of the economy has ceased; a long-term deflation follows. Buyers have greater advantage than sellers, and public opinion becomes more influential. The disparities in income widen and the poverty of the citizens is accelerated, bringing about dissatisfaction with the political and the economic system.

British people had negative feelings against the EU's bureaucratic control.

•Prime Minister Theresa May of the UK gave a speech after a meeting with President Trump, stating that the era of the United States and the UK being the prime world movers together has passed.

•The number of refugees may also increase in China and North Korea.

•The US has ceased to be the world's police force, and has adopted an "America first" way of thinking. Part of the reason for this is because many people think that, because so many countries possess nuclear weapons, the era of there being no long-standing wars will continue. No major wars will erupt because of the threat posed by the nuclear weapons. The United States has succeeded in producing shale oil, decreasing their reliance on the Middle East and other oil-producing regions.

•The US budget deficit continues to grow, weakening the country's economic vitality.

•The recovery of domestic manufacturing capacity in the US, the reduction of taxes, an increase in infrastructure investment, and the higher import tariffs proposed by the Trump administration will not necessarily lead to the recovery of the US economy. The future policies of the United States will most likely worsen the economic situations of China and Russia. Economic trends in China will become the focus of the world from now on. The collapse of the economy will lead to the collapse of the political systems.

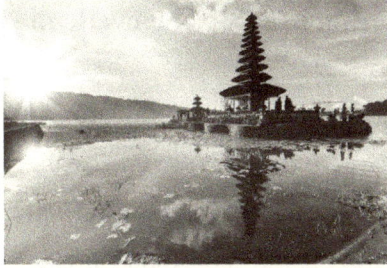

CHAPTER TWO

Material civilization will eventually fall apart in the future. The products of all industries will turn to dust. The agricultural industry will become the main industry for the new civilization.

1. The Earth is influenced by the cyclic movement of the Zodiac.

Because of the axial tilt of the Earth, stars in Zodiac change their position over the course of a 26,000 year cycle.

Coinciding with reversals in this cycle, the continents of Mu, Lemuria and Atlantis sank. The materialism of the civilization at that time brought about the collapse of the bubble economy. This civilization produced zero energy; the energy on earth was all consumed in the rise of this materialistic civilization. Because of the energy that was lost, the north pole tilted south and the continents in the northern hemisphere shifted due to the unbalanced distribution of dry land to the north. This process resulted in the poles shifting, which caused the magnetic reversal of north and south. This was the reason for the collapse of these three civilizations. The sea became land, and the land became sea.

Nobody predicted the fall of the Berlin Wall. Now the United States and China have become two heavily indebted superpowers. They cannot repay the debt with their current level of economic strength. With Brexit, it has become clear that the collapse of economies on both sides of the Dover Straits cannot be prevented. Deutsche Bank and other EU banks are in a state of insolvency.

In Russia, the ruble has depreciated by more than 60%, and domestic prices have risen. Pensioners are having a very hard time sustaining their livelihoods. When you look at Japan, people have experienced a 20-year-long deflation, and the economic growth witnessed by the previous generation has ceased. The capitalistic financial system is on the verge of falling apart.

In the 21st century, the material civilization focused on the industrious sector of industry will collapse and the agricultural industry will become the main one.

2. The industries of agriculture, animal husbandry, forestry, and fishery foster and encourage the growth of life.

People in the modern age are under the illusion that bodies and materials are all that life consists of, and take little account of the existence of spiritual life.

Dr. Einstein stated that all materials are made up of energy and mass. For human beings, these factors constitute life and body.

It is life (or the soul) that moves the body, sees and listens to things, and thinks. Modern science focuses on the external form of substances, as seen in quantum mechanics. All substances are subject to the law of entropy, and they are destined to disappear after beginning and ending. That the existence of atoms and electrons is immortal and cannot be destroyed.

Since human beings gain their knowledge from observing disappearing substances, the knowledge exists only temporarily, and can never be permanent.

The knowledge gained from disappearing substances is fake. It cannot be taken into the afterlife.

Wisdom comes from within. Because wisdom is also intuition, revelation, inspiration, and reality, you can take it with you even into the afterlife. And it can also accumulate.

Modern people value knowledge more than wisdom. It is obtained from substances. Substances consist of invisible atoms and electrons.

The substances are the result, and the atoms (oxygen) and electrons (hydrogen) are the cause. Laws exist that govern over atoms and electrons. God is the law that controls atoms and electrons. Human beings invented this God.

No matter how much we analyze the resultant substances, we do not know their causes. Even if we know through blood analysis that hepatic function is impaired, we do not know the cause.

The branch of science that researches the law that governs atoms and electrons and the discipline of causation is called space science. It is the science of the future.

It is said that physics and chemistry will not develop any further because these types of sciences only research into results.

3. The nature of the Earth has been destroyed over the past 40-50 years.

People cannot restore the natural environment because they do not know the cause of its destruction.

Because we do not know the cause of cancer, the treatment has consisted only in the removal of the cancer cells, or killing them with radiation or steroids.

The cause for cancer is that we break the laws that govern atoms (oxygen) and electrons (hydrogen).

When blood stagnation occurs, weaker parts of the body get damaged as blood continues to circulate around the healthy parts of the body. This is the cause of the intractable diseases of the present age.

The typical example is cancer.

It is necessary for us to reconstitute the stagnated blood and make it again healthily flowing blood. People seem not to understand what blood stagnation really means.

Oxygen is acidic, and hydrogen is alkaline. Modern science has produced only acidic chemical substances. As a result, we are surrounded by so many acidic substances; acid rain of PM 2.5 in the atmosphere, acidic food with the use of chemicals, acidic pharmaceutical products, and acidic radiation are a few examples. Nature essentially has a neutral charge. Modern science does not understand this fact.

A fetus is a bond of sperm (oxygen, acid) and an ovum (hydrogen, alkaline), which grows by cell division. Positive + negative = neutral. Oxygen + hydrogen = body. Mathematics in nature is oxygen 1 + hydrogen $1 = 1 \pm 0$ neutral. Humans are composed of atoms and electrons.

Nature is formed through integration and synthesis. 1 + 1 equals 1.

Dr. Einstein concluded that oxygen (energy) and hydrogen (mass) are in a relative relationship to one another, but in fact, it is correct to observe that they amalgamate with one another.

Nature always brings things back to neutral.

The natural environment is becoming more and more acidic because of human activities. To neutralize it, as nature tries to get rid of the acid it releases more acid to atmosphere. What happens then is that alkalinity increases, and makes things decompose and rot. The rotten state, wherein oxygen deficiency leads to destruction in nature, is the same as the condition of someone who has an intractable disease.

Acid is oxygen, alkaline is hydrogen. Oxygen is a life energy, and hydrogen is a body.

The idea that radical oxygenation is the cause of cancer is not correct. In the age of the dinosaurs, 60% of the air was oxygen (40% of the original radical oxygen O_1 + 20% of the O_2).

With the impact of meteorites, the 40% of O_1 was burned off, and only O_2 survived. Massive numbers of animals and plants became extinct and only smaller organisms could survive.

Humans, plants, and animals are aggregates of water. Dissolved oxygen becomes aerobic bacteria in water.

These bacteria like oxygen, and create it by means of photosynthesis. These are male bacteria. The bacteria that do not like oxygen but hydrogen are called the anaerobic bacteria i.e. female bacteria. Most microbiology societies do not understand the function of these male and female bacteria.

Functions of bacteria

	(1) When balanced - Marriage /nurturing / good bacillus	When unbalanced Separation / illness / bad bacteria	
Aerobic bacteria (O_2) - male Anaerobic bacteria (H) - female	Compose, grow Compose, grow	Dispersal · escape Dispersal · rot · disease	When aerobic bacteria are brought back, return to (1) balanced state → disease gets cured

....

When a man and a woman pair up, they marry and create children. The man is acidic and the woman is alkaline. The male/aerobic bacteria carry oxygen, favor acidity, air and light; the female/anaerobic bacteria favor hydrogen, darkness and water. They also prefer alkalinity.

*Nature balances (harmonizes). Plants grow in harmonized conditions where well-balanced light and darkness, air and water and aerobic bacteria and anaerobic bacteria are available.

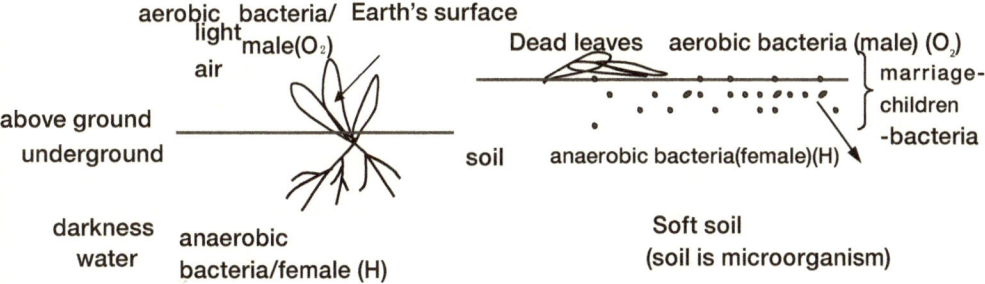

aerobic bacteria/ Earth's surface
light male(O_2)
air

above ground
underground

darkness
water

anaerobic
bacteria/female (H)

Dead leaves   aerobic bacteria (male) (O_2)
marriage-
children
-bacteria

soil   anaerobic bacteria(female)(H)

Soft soil
(soil is microorganism)

As shown in the diagram, the natural world is + and -,or the male and the female pair that maintain the neutral state.

Modern science does not understand this. It produces acidic chemicals and continues to use strongly acidic radioactivity.

The soil is the child of bacteria. We say that we should make soil, but only bacteria are capable of making soil. We kill these bacteria with pesticides and herbicides. It is terrible science.

4. A problem of the present age: Not knowing that microorganisms are vitally important in the natural world, we are killing them as "germs"

Space is full of microorganisms. Because it is vacuous space, even light and radio waves do not go through it.

Microorganisms also have pairs of male and female. As they are male (O_2) and female (H), H_2O (water vapor) is also present. The air, the water and the soil are all filled with a group of microorganisms.

Microorganisms are elementary particles. They permeate the whole universe and the natural world. When pesticide kills microorganisms in the air, the part with no microorganisms becomes an air pocket, therefore an airplane can go down to the ground because the lifting force is gone.

Migratory birds also go down to the ground. The human body has 6 billion cells and the number of bacteria reaches 8000 trillion. Minerals are aggregates of dead bacteria. Plants and animals are also aggregates of bacteria. Water is as well. When electronically disintegrated, it is divided into acidic water and alkaline water. This happens because it is divided into oxygen, which creates aerobic bacteria, and hydrogen, which creates anaerobic bacteria.

Building up the blood, flesh and bones in the body is also the work of microorganisms.

However, humans are killing these microorganisms as germs. For that reason, microorganisms have begun to attack back at mankind. The spread of the infection O - 157 among people is the beginning of the attack.

The most notorious natural destruction is desertification and the destruction of the natural environment in big cities.

New destructive viruses are emerging here. There is no drug to cure them.

Abnormalities of microorganisms can be found all over the world, as well as in Japan.

Organic zinc facilitates the growth of large livestock and vegetables, but chemical companies have developed chemicals that can act as female hormones in animals or plants. Gibberellin and cytokinin are used to grow large livestock and vegetables. If young boys up to the age of junior high school students eat those meat and vegetables, their sperm count will be reduced, due to the female hormones contained in those foods. They start to develop enlarged breasts and other feminine features. Even after they grow into adults, it is a big worry whether they can produce descendants or not because of their reduced number of sperm. This is the biggest problem with environmental hormones. We know that there are many kinds of plants that contain organic zinc. Global Family has developed a growth stimulant for livestock and vegetables that contains organic zinc.

People may think that you cannot grow vegetables without the use of agrochemicals, but we have set a record of growing rice without any agrochemicals for 13 consecutive years. Similar records have been achieved all over the country. The taste appraisal value of such rice is also 100 percent, which is the highest.

Intractable diseases among cattle, much like human's, such as cancer, pneumonia, and leukemia all have been cured.

Nutrition and energy from the food consumed by humans and livestock animals are absorbed through the wall of the intestine. But it is also true that Escherichia coli and bifidobacteria in the large intestine eat and disintegrate the remaining food so that it can be discharged as feces.

Bacteria repeat the cycle of birth, death and rebirth. They propagate themselves by eating the food that humans have eaten. The intestine absorbs the dead bacteria as nutrients. Similarly, the roots of plants absorb the dead bacteria in the soil as nutrients. Dead bacteria are the organic matter in the soil. Dead bacteria are white crystals of protein and minerals.

Modern agriculture is massively killing off bacteria in the soil and leaves with pesticides and herbicides. It kills microorganisms that grow plants, and provides inorganic fertilizer that microorganisms cannot eat. We are committing vandalism against nature by completely ignoring the rules of nature.

The law of nature is that malnourished plants should not leave offspring. That is why we have insects.

However, humans assume that the insect is the culprit, and give the plants stronger pesticides. Insects will increase their number of eggs. Eventually we will have an insect plague. We must realize that nature always overrides humans.

Modern science has come to a dead end. It is time for us to reflect, realize and appreciate the law of nature. We should once again acknowledge that things that are visible are composed of invisible units. And we must understand what laws govern those invisible atoms (oxygen) and electrons (hydrogen), and how microorganisms work.

5. Unknown function of microorganisms (bacteria)

Microorganisms build up blood, flesh and bone at room temperature in about 3 minutes. This is called biological transmutation.

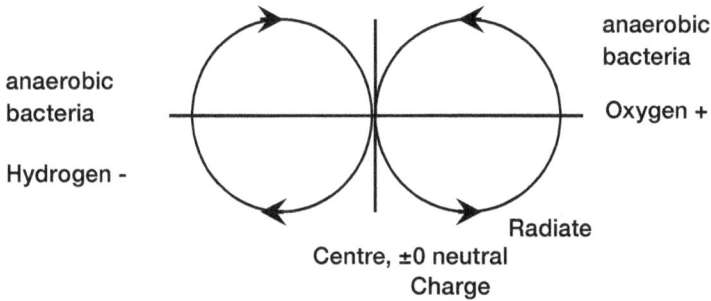

When male bacteria (O_2) and female (H) pair up and stay in balance, the central charge is neutral, ± 0, and two rotational motions of light start at the center. The fastest rotation speed in nature is 1.86 trillion times per second. At this speed, the atoms and electrons bond together, and increase the number of electrons available to create matter. This is called the transmutation of elements at normal temperature. Unless you understand the principal that lies behind the generation of light energy, we cannot start engaging in a scientific inquiry. Circular movement takes place on a continuous track. It is infinite movement.

The blood, flesh and bones in the body are formed at room temperature in 3 minutes. This rotational movement is called the Moebius ring in the Western society, and in Japan it is called Ashikabi circulation or Hyotan kara Koma (something very unexpected can come out of something ordinary). All of these terms mean the creation of new matter.

This process is common in humans, animals, and plants. IPS cells were developed without this notion, though the Nobel Prize was given for research into this type of cells.

It says in the Bible, 'Your kingdom come, your will be done, on earth as it is in heaven,' indicating that we should apply the technique of normal-temperature element transmutation and put it in practice.

Microorganisms have different sizes. Ordinary-sized bacteria in nature can be seen under a microscope at a rate of magnification of 800x. There are also other bacteria that can be seen only under an electron microscope. Infinitesimal microorganism that cannot be seen also exist. In fact, what called elementary particles are also bacteria. Bacteria of various sizes exist.

Bacteria are completely reading people's minds. In the life of bacteria as a group, the rules of coexistence, symbiosis, mutual aid and sharing apply to them. Bacteria do not fight each other. However, humans do fight and act selfishly. Bacteria may mimic human beings. Considering that humans may at times go off on their own, some bacteria will isolate themselves from the organization of the group. Those bacteria will go on to decay, because they become unable to function as parts of the group. With the intention to survive by themselves, they also may begin to eat the cell next to them and thereby grow bigger. Both become cancer cells. They decay.

Suppose you are fermenting bacteria. Because bacteria are reading your mind, if you are selfish and radiating rough vibrations, then the bacteria will disagree with you. The bacteria turn away and do not ferment. If you finely cut the leaves of a branch using a mechanical trimmer, you also kill or hurt the bacteria with the sharp blades. The bacteria will get angry and will decide not ferment. Fermentation becomes complete when the number of bacteria increases by 1000 times.

Since vibrations vary from person to person, there are as many kinds of fermentation as numbers of people. Birds of a feather flock together. The bacteria react to the difference in vibration.

Species-specific bacteria inhabit every plant. Banana leaves contain bacteria specific for bananas, just as radish leaves have radish bacteria. Bacteria specific for ginseng leaves inhabit ginseng, creating saponins, amino acids and minerals. If you let ginseng bacteria and cordyceps sinensis bacteria live in spinach leaves, the bacteria of all three plants will coexist and produce the medicinal properties of herbs. You can easily produce spinach with medicinal properties that are as potent as those found in ginseng or cordyceps. Everyone can make food that can be a medicinal source.

Genetic modification is not necessary at all.

Bacteria help to form the bodies of plants, animals, and humans, by means of biological transmutation.

Unless these elements are organic, they cannot be separated into atoms and electrons. Unless the minerals it receives are organic, the human body cannot convert them into blood, flesh or bone. The minerals in mineral water cannot be absorbed into the body because they are inorganic.

Drip infusion into the human body contains inorganic minerals, so the minerals do not become blood, flesh or bone. People fertilize soil with inorganic nitrogen, phosphorus or potassium, but because the bacteria in the soil do not eat inorganic matter, these fertilizers do not nourish the soil.

Modern science ignores the process of element transformation. If it ignores this process, they should not call it science. Scientists do not understand the function of microorganisms. Modern science is not natural science. Microorganisms should play the leading role in agriculture, animal husbandry and medicine. A living organism is an aggregate of cells.

How does a cell work?

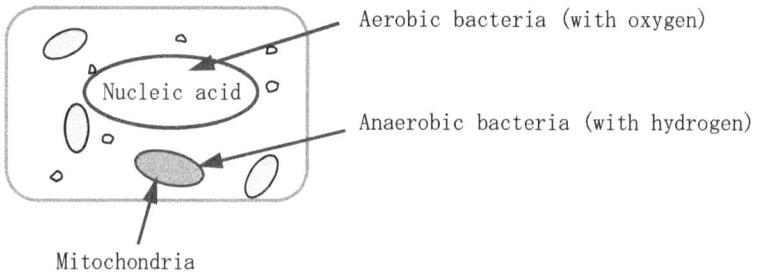

Aerobic bacteria (with oxygen)

Nucleic acid

Anaerobic bacteria (with hydrogen)

Mitochondria

Aerobic bacteria and oxygen inhabit Nucleic acids, and anaerobic bacteria and hydrogen inhabit the surroundings.

When oxygen and hydrogen are balanced and harmonized, the center becomes ± 0, with a neutral charge, and two rotational motions of light start from there.

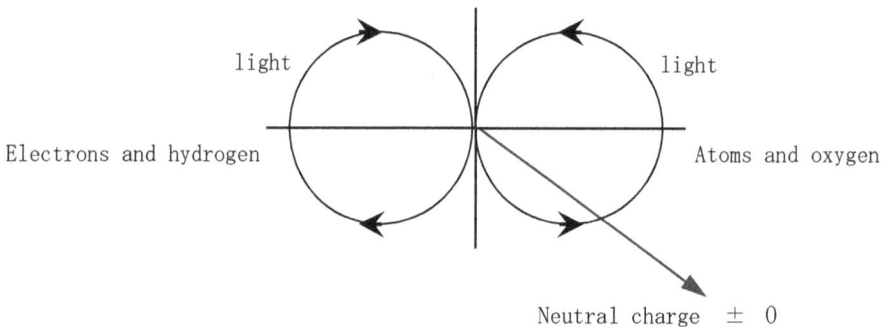

light

light

Electrons and hydrogen

Atoms and oxygen

Neutral charge ± 0

Cells are light energy generators. In a scientific dictionary, the amount of electricity generated by each part of human body is shown as XX mV (millivolt). We have electric energy.

Cells function as batteries. Even if one cell only generates 1.5 volts, that would be 9 billion volts coming from 6 billion cells. The cell produces infinite energy.

Pairs of oxygen-carrying microorganisms and hydrogen-carrying microorganisms exist in space, and each one of them is generating 1.5-2 volts. Since the number of microorganisms is infinite, it can be said that we are surrounded by infinite cosmic energy.

The complete balance of + and − was referred to by Buddha as moderation, the middle way, mercy. Jesus called it love. Love does not mean to like or to dislike. What it means is complete harmony. Buddha called it moderation, the middle way, or mercy.

All living organisms are the aggregate of cells. Cells will start to generate light energy when the neutral charge is achieved by + and −. People call this aura.

When you learn about and believe in the balance of life between the mind and the body, which is the notion that your essence is in life, especially in space life, you will generate an aura. That is because you have greater energy. Comprehensive amino acids and comprehensive minerals are necessary to grow healthy cells. Both plants and animals are aggregates of cells, aggregates of microorganisms. In order to activate cells, we need to create a neutral environment.

There are over 400 kinds of amino acids in nature. There are over 70 kinds of minerals as well. People think that they only need between 6 and 12 kinds of essential amino acids. Of the 70 kinds of minerals, only nitrogen, phosphorus and potassium are put in vegetables, and those are inorganic minerals.

There are also 5 to 6 kinds of minerals added to drip infusions for humans, but because they are also inorganic, they cannot be absorbed and people become malnourished. To activate the cells of animals and plants, it is better to give them comprehensive amino acids and minerals as nourishment. The taste of the cells also improves.

In order to improve the taste of rice, an effective technique is to provide amino acids as fertilizers. Just a small amount of organic minerals has the power to cure intractable diseases.

Germanium and selenium bring oxygen. This process can cure intractable diseases. Lithium will strengthen the white blood cells. Vanadium improves blood flow.

These organic minerals are produced as the output of microorganisms that undergo elemental transmutation. Organic zinc is the most effective of all minerals that promote natural growth.

In the world of microorganisms, there are bacteria that have survived for billions of years after having created the earth's resources. Now, we can utilize them. Cyanobacteria and *Haematococcus pluvialis* bacteria supplied oxygen to the earth between 2 billion to 3 billion years ago. By photosynthesis, they can supply more than 200 times as much oxygen as ordinary land plants can. Using the oxygen supplied by cyanobacteria and *Haematococcus pluvialis* bacteria, a portion of a rice field was revitalized and aquatic biota such as Japanese rice-fish, pond snails, pond loach and fireflies were able to return in just a few months. These are the best plants for restoring destroyed natural environments.

When you ingest the fermented solution of bacteria, the blood flow through the capillaries improves in no time, assisting the function of your brain and eyes. Also, energy flow in the spine improves, and the body's natural healing power and immunity will improve. Iron-oxidizing bacteria, which produce iron, can be used to warm soil and greenhouses. Because it is an organic iron, it strengthens the body.

If you soak a cloth with a dyeing solution rich in iron-oxidizing bacteria, you can use this cloth to cover yourself and it will keep you warm as well as make the microorganism and cells in your body more active.

Since the microorganisms that live in the leaves of herbs have unique amino acids, minerals, and medicinal properties, if you can increase these microorganisms and ingest them, you would no longer need chemicals and could get much greater benefit from medicinal herbs.

Shennong (an agricultural god), an ancient medicine god of China, is said to have written the Shennong Bencaojing (The Classic of Herbal Medicine). He classified herbs into three categories; 'noble' or 'higher herbs;' 'human', 'common,' or 'middle herbs;' and 'lower herbs.' It is said that the higher herbs are all-purpose drugs that are free from adverse effects. If you take them for a long time you can be like a god or the hermits.

Medicinal herbs are always accompanied by unique spirits. Because they are higher discarnate-entities, they have omnipotent wisdom. They will heal the stress in people's minds.

List of the effects of useful vegetable bacteria

Revised in 2016.9

1	Decomposing type	Sugarcane, Papaya, Pineapple, Stevia
2	Cooling and moisturizing	Sugarcane
3	Enzyme making	Papaya
4	Nitrogen absorption	Soybeans, Red bean, Ginnem tree

5	Generation of oxygen	Cyanobacteria
	• mass production	Cyanobacteria, *Haematococcus pluvialis,* Arthrospira
	• low temperature	Snow lotus
	• Vitamin C	Amla (or indian gooseberry)
6	Production of beta carotene	*Haematococcus pluvialis*
7	Decomposition of radioactive matter	Sunflower, *Aspergillus oryzae* ('Koji' mold)
8	Decomposition of heavy metal	Sunflower, Holy basil
9	Decomposition of mercury	Holy basil
10	Salt decomposition	Seaweed, Isomatsu *(Limonium wrightii var. arbusculum)*
11	Oil decomposition	Pine, Oil digesting enzymes, Sunflower
12	High in amino acid (especially lysine)	Amaranthus (0.8 mg / 100 g), Sea buckthorn (68), Maca (55), Undiluted black vinegar (120), Cordyceps militaris (980), head and bony parts of bonito (500), Borojo (200)
13	High in calcium	Amaranthus (152mg / 100g), Rawan butterbur (1600), Maca (220), Giant Kelp (2000), Sesame meal (1200), *Bidens pilosa* (1800), Drumstick tree (Moringa oleifera) (3087)
14	zinc	Maca (2.8mg / 100g), Giant Kelp (6.6), Sesame meal (7.1), Bidens pilosa (6.7), giant ragweed (400)
15	Detoxification	Sunflower, Coptis japonica (from Sichuan), gold-and-silver honeysuckle, octopus bush (habu Trimeresurus flavoviridis poisoning), *Echinacea,* Japanese knotweed, holy basil, Kuding Tea, Root of wild *Polygonum Multiflorum* (tuber fleeceflower), Pollen, Lotus, Broadleaf cattail
16	Antiviral, antimicrobial	Propolis, Shell ginger, Neem, Sophora root, Wasabi, Tropical milkweed, Pollen, Teatree, Holy basil Fermented solution with pH 3 or less - Snow lotus, Amla (Indian gooseberry)

17	Organic germanium	Wild Reishi mushroom
18	intuition, revelation, inspiration	Ayahuasca, San Pedro cactus, Peyote, Yarrow, St. John's Wort, common vervain, orange day-lily, *Cordyceps militaris*, Xylaria nigripes, Psilocybin mushrooms
19	Other minerals	
	• germanium	Reishi (1000mg / 100g), *Heterochordaria abietina* 'sea fir' (1800)
	• phosphorus	Dried *Sergia lucens* (1200mg / 100g), dried banded blue sprat (1200)
	• vanadium	vanadium（20000mg／100g)
20	Calming	Chaga mushroom, St. John's wort, Jujube, tuber fleeceflower, *Atractylodes japonica*, agnolia vine, pseudobulb of *Cremastra appendiculata (D.Don) Makino*, Poria, Maca
21	Stomachic effects	American Silvertop, Medicated Leaven, *Agrimonia pilosa*, Myohakuboku *Atractylodes japonica*
22	Vasodilatation	*Cistanche tubulosa*, root of *Polygonum multiflorum* (tuber fleeceflower)
23	Mild alkalization of blood	Seeds of Japanese Loquat
24	Brain activity	*Cordyceps sinensis*, Snow lotus *(saussurea medusa)*, Ginseng, Pseudoginseng, Wuling Mushroom
25	Longevity	Reishi mushroom, Ginseng, *Panax notoginseng*, Snow lotus, Golden root, Himalayan Ginseng, *Laricifomes officinalis* (agarikon), Tongkat Ali, *Cistanche tubulosa*, Isomatsu *(Limonium wrightii var.arbusculum)*
26	Natural radioactivity	Gymnema
27	Pain relief	Snow lotus, Opium poppy, *Erythroxylum coca*, Cannabis, *Aconitum carmichaeli Gentiana scabra var. buergeri*, Axilla, Holy basil, Red yeast rice (Koji) , Tiger's bone

| 28 | Cholesterol decomposition | Pine pollen, Fu tea, Kuding Tea from 1000-year-old tree, Qing Shan Lu Shui tea, *Panax notoginseng*, Eucommia Tea, pollen, propolis, 1800-year-old tree Pu'er tea |
| 29 | tonic, blood flow improvement | Tongkat Ali, *Panax notoginseng*, *Cordyceps sinensis*, Maca, Ginseng |

Each herb has slightly different effects within the category.

I will show the function and the personality of the spirit, as well as the message from the spirit.

Spirit chooses people. Since the spirit can only abide in pure consciousness, the spirit will choose people who have reached the highest state of consciousness, who can understand the spirit. It will take those people along from the beginning. The spirits will lead you to find the essence of things. They take you as you are. There is no wall between the spirit and the person. The only difference is that you have a physical body and the spirit does not. The body deprives people of freedom. People are trapped in constraints. The spirit does not understand the physical level, because the body does not exist for the spirit. Physical illness is something people invented. When you notice the mistake that has been made, the disease disappears. What you need to do to get rid of an illness is to relax and release the mind. Please give prayers to the spirits. Please pray that the spirit will help you do the work of curing the disease. The spirit will work for you and guide you in the right direction when it feels you are doing the right thing. God has given it free will. When you listen to the voices of the spirit and resonate with them, you will be able to understand the joy of working together. Be peaceful. Pray for peace. Then you will be able to work with the spirit. -Message from the Spirit	Hemp It will help purify the body. It also has a calming effect, and the ability to adjust vibrations. It has the function of restoring cells to their normal condition. The hemp spirit is a shy spirit who is fond of taming people. Coca Motherly love, love of Pachamama. It removes all pain. It teaches love and forgiveness. The spirit of coca possesses gentleness, tolerance, pleasure, brightness, and greatness. A child of Pachamama lives in it. Chaparral The spirit of chaparral possesses greatness, tolerance, grandeur, cheerfulness, and masculine love. It leads you to expand your consciousness, and to have translucent consciousness. The chaparral spirit is the head of the spirits. Ayahuasca This plant has the power to purify the physical level and bring you back to the true self. By looking at the deeper consciousness, we can reach the essence of things. The spirit of honesty, humility, and purity lives here.

Recently, a seven-year-old boy in Hokkaido was dropped off from his father's car and went missing for six days but was found well and healthy. He walked throughout the night, until he found an abandoned house where he remained safe until he was discovered. He covered ground that was several times larger than the Tokyo Dome.

Children of today have been born as people of the 21st century. They have higher sensibilities than those who were born in the 20th century. This is why the current century will bring about the Utopian society. Children up to 12-years-old can see spirits and have conversations with them. Because the spirits are higher discarnate entities, they are omnipotent.

In the middle of the night, the spirits manifested as light bodies and illuminated the way so that the child was guided to a safe and unlocked building with water and mats. Every day the spirits and the child communicated with each other, and the child was found well on the sixth day. Adults do not understand this.

6. If you put plants in a place that has a neutral charge, the plants will have no stress and grow to be big and healthy.

All over the world, people put their hands together when they pray. Why do they do that? The right side of your body is positively charged, i.e. it is the N pole, the left side is negatively charged, i.e. it is the S pole. The region of the body above the navel is positively charged and the lower half of the body is negatively charged. When material civilization develops, the negative, or the legs, will develop to become longer. The right hand is the N pole, the left hand is the S pole and the middle is $\pm$ 0, i.e. neutral. Neutrality is the state of nature and of God, and the praying position represents this.

Ksitigarbha (the Buddhist deity known in Japanese as 'Jizo') shows his right palm in front of his chest, and puts out his left hand in front of him. He radiates light from the N pole in the right hand, and absorbs the light in the S pole in the left hand, and recreates the rotational movement of the light. In modern times, this rotational movement is called ion exchange movement.

In a neutral state, people and animals can relax, and plants grow to be big. Place a 10 yen coin and 1 yen coin respectively on the left and right side of a flowerpot. The copper contained in the 10 yen coin represents the cation, while the aluminum of the 1 yen is the anion. The middle of the pot has a neutral charge. Because the stress on the plant is taken away, the size of its roots triples.

Roots enjoy being in the darkness in the soil. White flowerpots make roots feel stressed. If you change a white pot for a black one, you can triple the root size. When copper wires are placed on one side of a field or greenhouse and aluminum wires on the other, the center becomes electrically neutral.

Below is a picture of an onion grown under the above-mentioned conditions. You can see how big it has grown.

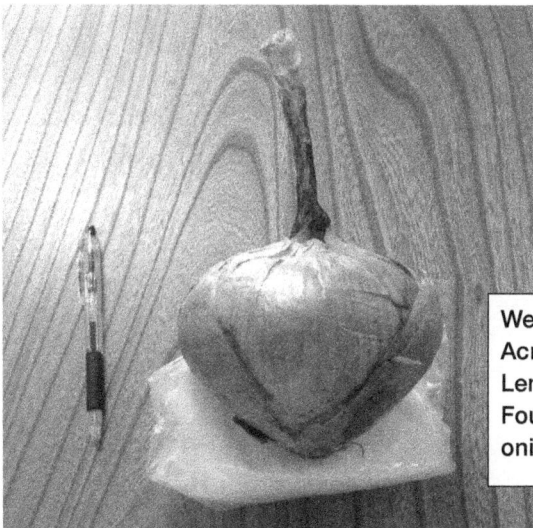

Weight: approx. 900 grams
Across: approx. 13cm
Length (the bulb) : approx.11cm
Four times larger than regular
onion (approx.200g)

If you neutralize a room by placing an aluminum panel on one side and a copper panel on the other, your body will feel relaxed.

$$- \quad \Box \quad +$$

Synthetic fibers are acidic. If you neutralize a room with alkaline water, the interior atmosphere becomes neutral and the body can rest.

Since concrete is acidic, if you build a house with concrete, your health will become damaged within 10 years. Neutralizing the concrete with strong alkaline water before it solidifies will cause it not to harm you and your family.

7. Why did the life-forms grow enormously during the dinasaur era?

Both plants and animals were huge but healthy in the age of the dinosaurs. There was a reason why they could grow so enormously. The submersion of the continents occurs in a 26,000-years cycle. Minerals from the land are drained into the sea by rain over this long period of time. Heavy minerals sink deep into the sea, more than 3000 meters below sea level. Light minerals also settle at the bottom of the sea at the same time. The deeper the sea is, the richer in minerals it becomes.

Also, plankton-derived amino acids are deposited on the deep ocean floor. When a seismic event occurs, the soil becomes very nutritious with abundant amino acids, minerals and microorganisms. That was why the plants grow enormously and release a large amount of oxygen through photosynthesis. The oxygen that is emitted is called O_1 oxygen, which is the original active form of oxygen that can help to grow things greatly. It has the characteristic of being half-way between O_2 and O_3. As O_1 oxygen then comprised 40% of the atmosphere, and O_2 was 20%, both plants and animals had a high amount of 60% of oxygen altogether in the atmosphere, enabling them to grow enormously. With the use of a simple device that converts O_2 to O_1, we can instantly obtain O_1 oxygen.

If you attach an O_1 oxygen conversion ring to the outlet of the air pump of an aquarium, the water becomes rich in O_1 oxygen. Small goldfish will grow to be very large, and the leaves of the aquatic plants will grow to more than twice their normal size.

This O_1 oxygen has a strong disinfectant capability. The fish in the aquarium grow big and germs do not develop. Fish food left uneaten does not rot.

Plants will grow huge in a short period of time if you feed your soil with organic minerals and amino acid fertilizers, spray a growth-promoting agent with organic zinc on the leaves, and add O_1 oxygen to the atmosphere. A water hyacinth grown under these conditions got to be three times as big as normal ones in a short period of time.

8. Develop the compost to grow huge plants ... They grow more than 4 times bigger

The Great Pyramid at Giza is a light energy generating device in which acidic rock (oxygen) and alkaline rock (hydrogen) are alternately stacked. The top is covered with white phosphate ore. Phosphorus has the property of igniting at 40°C, and has the function of helping the oxygen and hydrogen to generate light energy.

This is called the principle of 'Lin San Kali.' It means phosphorus, acid and alkali.

To carry out this process, we used three agricultural materials; one is strongly acidic, one is highly alkaline and the other is bone meal (phosphorus). They generated light energy. Using this energy, we succeeded in growing onions that are 4 times as big as normal ones.

Burdock grew to 3.2 kg in weight, with girth of 32 cm. If you search on YouTube for 'non-agrochemical burdock', you can see the video taken at the time of digging. I call this 'the pyramid compost.' It is easy to make.

When we used this type of compost on only a 991 m^2 section of a rice field in the Tsugaru region, all the rice in a field of 4462 m^2 grew longer by an average of 15 cm or more. Hollows in the soil allowed the light energy to spread all throughout the 4462 m^2 field. This pyramid compost can be called a new inorganic fertilizer. Neither damage from pests nor diseases have been reported. Migratory birds and wildlife gather in this rice field because of its strong energy.

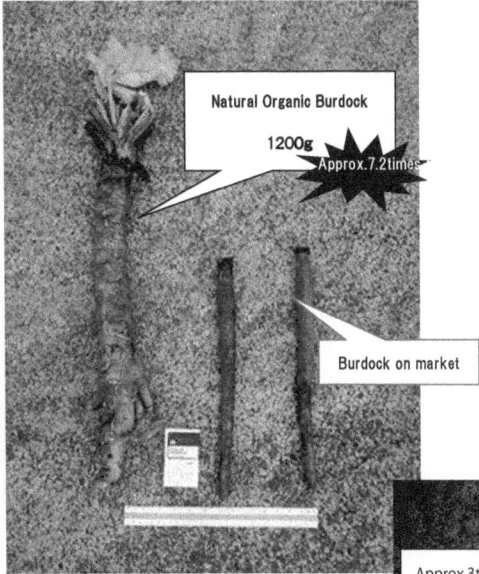

Natural Organic Burdock

1200g

Approx.7.2times

Burdock on market

Nov.18, 2010   Producer： Ikuko Kubo

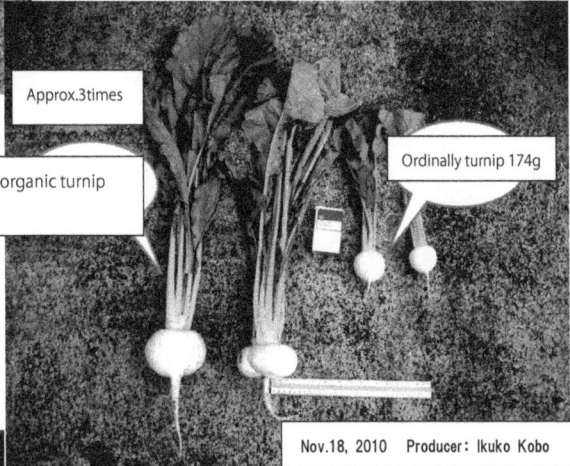

Approx.3times

Natural organic turnip

538g

Ordinally turnip 174g

Nov.18, 2010   Producer： Ikuko Kobo

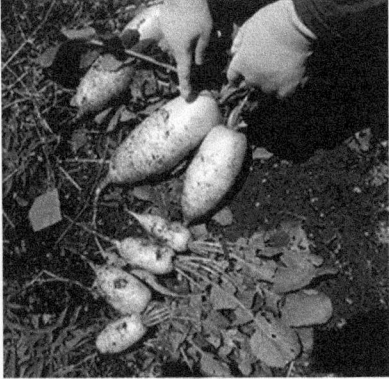

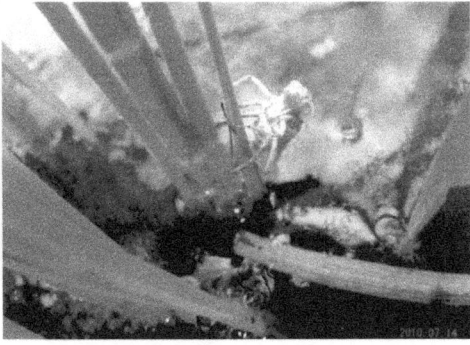

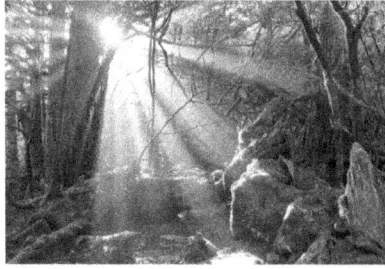

CHAPTER THREE

The art of agriculture is the cultivation of knowledge. Learn the law of the growth of vegetables.

1. Who takes care of growing plants?

① After rain, plants grow rapidly. Why?

Woods, forests, grass fields – They are all healthier than the vegetables grown in vegetable patches. Why is that?

② What are the roles played by the sun and the moon?

Which is best suited for sowing seeds, a new moon or a full moon? When is the best time for harvesting watermelons or tomatoes? Modern people have forgotten these things.

③ We need the four major elements that promote the growth of life in nature on earth:

Earth, water, fire, air. What role do they play?

If any of the soil, water, fire or the air are contaminated, living creatures, including human beings, cannot survive.

④ Microorganisms assist the growth of plants, humans, animals and minerals.

The remains of microorganisms become fertilizer for plants to absorb by their roots. This means that plants consist of organic matter.

Microorganisms living in leaves change CO_2 to O_2 through photosynthesis.

The protein that was contained in the remains of bacteria is made into amino acid. Microorganisms in leaves produce amino acid and minerals that have the medicinal properties unique to that plant.

Modern science does not recognize the role of

microorganisms. Scientists kill them as germs.

⑤ Why do clouds develop? Why does it rain? They are supported by plants.

Tree roots can hold 1-2 tons of water in them. On the other hand, leaves evaporate water so that they can keep themselves cool in the heat of the sun. Water vapor from leaves develops into and becomes clouds and rain. Thanks to this water, roots can live to support branches and leaves, and flowers can bloom. If people cut down large numbers of trees, the land will not get as much rainfall, and this makes the land dryer. Drought takes place. This is the destruction of nature.

2. Understand the meaning of the "Tree of Life" and "sakaki" tree *(Cleyera japonica).*

You might have seen the picture of the Tree of Life from the Mayan civilization. Let's think here about the meaning of the "sakaki tree" in Japanese Shintoism.

Because there are roots, a tree can have a trunk and branches. Because there are branches the tree can have leaves. Roots-Branches-Leaves-Vapor connect the earth to the heavens. Every leaf derives from one tree, and this means that each has a life of equal value to any other. Because human lives also consist of energy and mass, we can say there is only one kind of unlimited energy in the entire universe. The Tree of Life and sakaki tree indicate that everything on the earth is made to live by the life force of the universe.

The being that governs all lives and the lives that are made to live by that being are all interconnected.

In order for any life to exist, there must be some existence enabling that life to live. There is only one life force in the entire universe. The spiritual branches of life in the universe are minerals, plants, animals and humans. There exists only the Creator and His branches. People may think that the world is made up of two existences; those that are made to live and the Creator who gives them life. However, it is in fact monogenesis. Cause and effect converge into one. They are two sides of the same coin. The Tree of Life and sakaki tree show us that.

Both visible substances and the invisible entities that exist as energy bodies are one.

Visible matter is formed by oxygen (positive ions, atoms) and hydrogen (negative ions, electrons), which are invisible. The aggregate of invisible microorganisms becomes visible substance.

Higher discarnate entities and lower discarnate entities are both branches of the Creator's Universal consciousness. The only difference is that one type of being is at the developmental stage, and the other being is close to completion.

Everything is connected as one. Consciousness and life are the same.

Therefore, they are supposed to be able to talk to each other. This is called telepathy, or thought transference. Animals, plants, minerals and microorganisms can communicate to each other, as they all source from the same life energy

If you tell your vegetables that you love them six times a day, they grow three to four times larger than vegetables grown ordinarily. If you establish heart-to-heart communication with your livestock, such that the animal and you feel that you belong to the same life force, and smile to them, then they understand and accept you. We can understand each other.

Agricultural industry deals with everything that has life.

Microorganisms live in a group, and as I mentioned before, they live under the rule of coexistence and symbiosis, with the spirit of mutual aid and sharing. If you are irritated, microorganisms will not want to cooperate with you, and you will not be able to achieve good fermentation. Microorganisms can read your mind 100%. There are just so many people who do not know this principle.

3. Root cause analysis of decreased plant growth

Modern agriculture is not only starving microorganisms but even killing them with agrochemicals and pesticides. Microorganisms that could be the food for plant roots have all died out.

People have been ignoring for a long time the fact that killing ants means killing people.

Ants dig tunnels in the ground and bring oxygen into the earth.

With this oxygen, worms and moles can live and eliminate waste. Their waste comprises the mass of microorganisms that can feed microorganisms. Edaphon increases and the soil becomes nutritious for plants. If you kill ants with pesticides, the plants die. Nature runs in cycles. Roots feed on the decaying bodies of microorganisms.

In China, farmers only use chemical fertilizers without giving any food to the microorganisms. Therefore, microorganisms in the soil cannot survive. Microorganisms usually collect water, so without microorganisms, the soil becomes dry and hard, or turns to desert and gets blown away by the wind. The land dies.

On top of that, water is being misused for industrial purposes and becomes contaminated. At times, water from the Yellow River does not flow into the ocean for many days. Such a water shortage for agriculture has caused the farmland to dry out.

Now that the Chinese government has decided to abolish the

one-child policy, the population has started growing again, and the shortage of food has become a serious problem.

Modern agriculture kills the microorganisms in the soil and the leaves. The plants suffer malnutrition, making them susceptible to pests, like insects. This type of agriculture destroys the natural environment.

People have begun introducing microorganisms into agriculture, but as they do not know how microorganisms work, the process is incomplete.

I would like to chronicle how people have come to be this way, and point out the problems we have now.

① *In the beginning...*
Organic farming: Pioneering the wilderness – Soil was completely nutritious for periods of three years – no need to worry about pests and weeds
Slash-and-burn farming: Soil was completely nutritious for two years - no need to worry about pests and weeds
Fallow farmland: Let weeds grow on 2/3 of the land for the soil to regain nutrients

↓

Humanure compost: Many years ago, people would deposit human waste in their farmland as manure after harvest.

② *Widespread use of synthetic fertilizers*

Synthetic fertilizers=inorganic fertilizers ...... these do not become food for edaphon

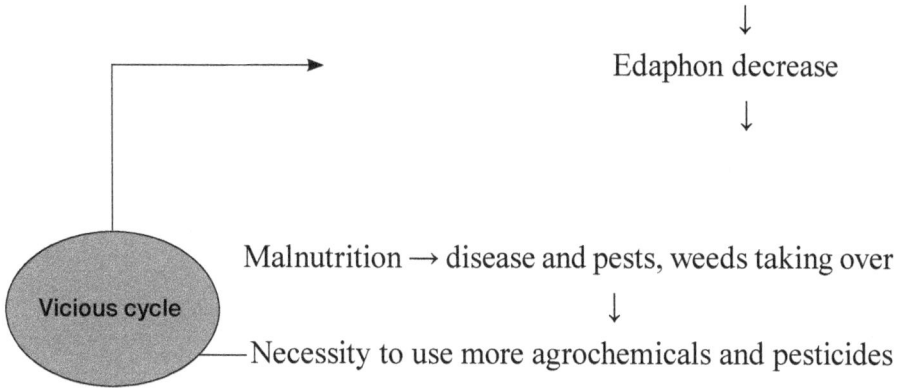

↓

Edaphon decrease

↓

Malnutrition → disease and pests, weeds taking over

↓

Necessity to use more agrochemicals and pesticides

Vicious cycle

Agrochemicals bring about pathogenic bacteria and pests with higher resistance to pesticides.

Pests produce more eggs, causing a plague of pests.

↓

Use of poisonous agrochemicals increases; the strength of the poison intensifies.

↓

Strongly acidic agrochemicals needed to kill stronger pests.

↓

Acidification of human body → Organs being damaged (break down, rot, melt)

↓

· Cancer, atopic dermatitis, bones and muscles lose thickness (due to lack of calcium) → killing people

· People become more irritated, hysterical, short-tempered – conflict, disorder → terrorism, war

③ *Need for organic farming*

Finding no edaphon → Burying untreated organic matter in the soil → Without enough bacteria, organic matter left unbroken down then goes to rot → Vegetables go rotten because of that → Incremental increase of disease and pests

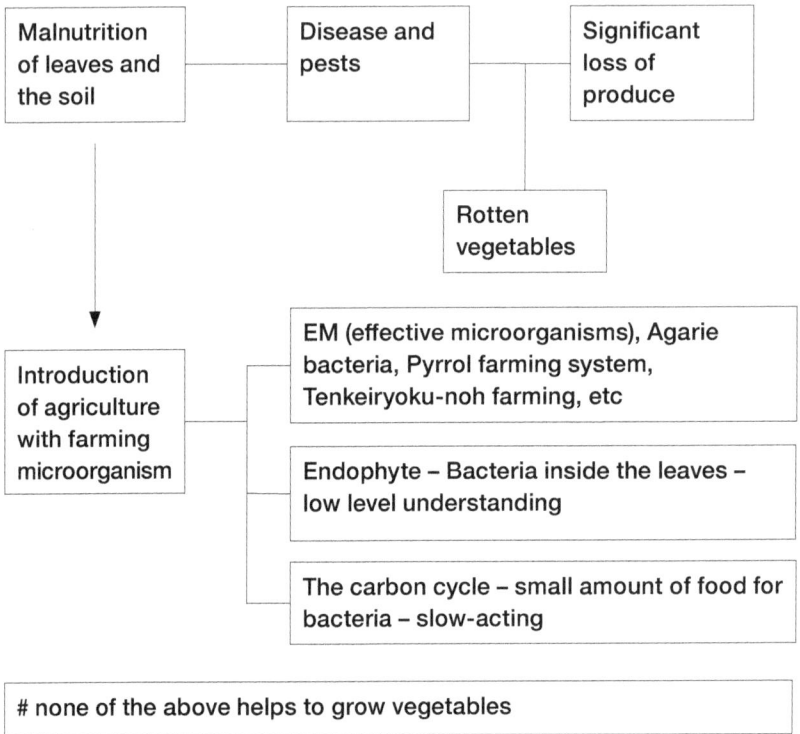

Malnutrition of leaves and the soil	Disease and pests	Significant loss of produce

Rotten vegetables

Introduction of agriculture with farming microorganism

- EM (effective microorganisms), Agarie bacteria, Pyrrol farming system, Tenkeiryoku-noh farming, etc
- Endophyte – Bacteria inside the leaves – low level understanding
- The carbon cycle – small amount of food for bacteria – slow-acting

none of the above helps to grow vegetables

↓

Diseases and pests – one type of edaphon – Side effects are that vegetables become rotten in the soil within three years

• Bacteria from Okinawa cannot function in areas north of Kansai because of the colder climate

↓

Ignorance of the natural processes of microorganisms
The carbon cycle, endophyte, EM, other microorganism farming products, photosynthetic bacteria, etc. – Oxygen, Hydrogen, Carbon - all of them are the basis of agriculture.

↓

The Beginning of Natural Farming

4. New natural farming

"Global Family" has developed a new natural farming method and begun spreading it all over Japan.

This method utilizes a combination of organic fertilizers (with effective microorganisms) and inorganic fertilizers (growing massive vegetables by generating light energy). There is no usage of agrochemicals whatsoever, yet there is no disease nor depletion of the soil year after year. Anyone can produce vegetables with medicinal properties that are as potent as those found in ginseng or cordyceps. It is very easy and does not cost much.

Liquid soil improver: A fermented liquid complex of multi-amino acids and multi-minerals that detoxify the soil from agricultural chemicals or dioxins. Radioactivity and heavy metals such as mercury break down. However long you have been using chemicals on your soil, our soil improver will make your farmland be free of any traces of chemicals in one month. Radioactivity will be broken down. Light energy will be generated in the soil. Everything will be neutralized and toxins will be rendered innocuous.

A farm in Asaka city, Saitama Prefecture grows carrots in their farmland of 660m^2 using natural farming methods. They certainly do not use any agrochemicals.

Next to this farmland is a newly opened McDonald's restaurant. The number of customers has increased rapidly and the restaurant achieved Number One in sales in the country within two years.

Because of the light energy generated by our liquid soil improver, customers started feeling good and pleasant. People also started noticing that their headaches went away.

If you feel good, you tend to stay at a place longer, and that is why the restaurant boosted its sales.

In winter, however, the number of customers who visit McDonald's goes back to normal, because the farm does not sprinkle the liquid soil improver.

Convenience stores and warehouses all increased their customer volumes.

Because of the higher energy levels, wild life, red dragonflies and other insects started to gather around the farmland.

Complete nutrition: This means concentrated fertilizers with multi-amino acids and multi-minerals that grow crops and vegetables very large and healthy, with their cells almost bursting.

The taste appraisal value of rice is measured by a taste analyzer. The national average is around 65-70 points, but the rice grown with natural farming methods scored 93 points on average and even 100 points at times. Testing of over 200 types of remaining chemicals showed that there were no chemicals detected. When we scored 93 points in tasting appraisal value, Mitsukoshi and Takashimaya, both long-established department stores in Japan, offered that they wished to sell our rice in their stores.

There lived a rice farmer and his wife in Aomori Prefecture who had rice fields of 178,500m^2 that used to produce only 180kg/990m^2 of low quality rice, which the farmers' union (JA) refused to purchase one year. After applying the natural farming method with the approval of the JA the following year, the same rice field produced 450kg/990m^2 of rice that was classified as first grade by the JA. They had fireflies in the rice field for the first time in 13 years.

The couple used to spend 1.2 million yen/year on weeding labor, but with the introduction of the natural farming method, the expenditure has gone down to zero in two years.

The husband says, "I come to the rice field every day to charge myself with the energy from the microorganisms in the rice field. This is the best farming I have ever known. My colleagues travel abroad in the off-season, but my wife and I would not wish to go to any foreign countries."

People at JA affirm that the husband's personality has changed.

One year in Shiga prefecture, they had a poor crop of rice. However, the rice field that used the natural farming method managed to produce healthy and tasty rice.

In Wadomari Town in Kagoshima Prefecture, the natural farming method has been the certified farming method of the town office and the JA for more than ten years. The town office ferments the liquid soil improver and sells it for 100yen/10l to farmers.

One year, there was an epidemic of disease from a virus that affected potatoes, and many potato farmers could not make any shipments. But the farmers who applied the natural farming method could ship their potatoes without any trouble.

They have been producing potatoes entirely without the use of agrochemicals.

5. Microorganisms play the leading part in natural farming, their fermentation and revolution.

Most people use incorrect methods of fermentation, which is the process of increasing the number of microorganisms. They make compost but because they do not know of any better fermentation method, it sometimes takes six months, or two weeks at the fastest.

We have developed a method to complete the fermentation process in two hours. You can increase seed bacteria 1000 times in two hours.

If you keep fermenting for another two hours, another 1000 times the number of bacteria will equal 1 million times. In another two hours you can have 1 billion bacteria.

You can have an eternal supply of bacteria. Easy. Low cost.

When light energy is generated, you can gather limitless energy that can be used as electricity. That is why we call this energy "free energy."

Male and female microorganisms, or pyramid composting, is free energy in itself.

Some people fight over water, but rain falls from the sky. When you cool down water vapor, you get water. Water vapor is limitless. The water supply is limitless.

The 21st century has seen the advent of many technologies that can supply things limitlessly. You do not need to spend a great deal of money.

The size of microorganisms and bacteria are usually 0.1micron. The same size as molecules in the air, or smoke. If you feed these bacteria with a few centimeters worth of food waste, they cannot eat it. It is as if you gave a person a whole watermelon, which of course would be impossible for him to eat. Bacteria starve to death.

However, bacteria can drink water. Brown sugar dissolves in

water. When you feed bacteria with food in the form of water, the number of bacteria multiplies within seconds.

A warmer environment accelerates the fermentation process.

When you try to increase bacteria, it is essential to feed them with something sweet as well as organic minerals. The best food would be the least processed raw brown sugar or rice bran. Powdered seaweeds are also organic minerals.

Bacteria found in nature cannot survive at temperatures under -30°C or above 130°C. They are alive at 100°C. However, viruses and germs die at 60°C.

Under 80°C, bacteria increase 1000 times in two hours and ferment completely.

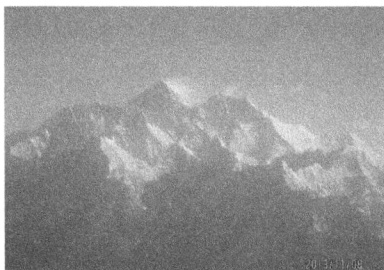

CHAPTER FOUR

The factors for plant growth

1. Why do plants grow rapidly after a rainfall?

Rain contains 79% nitrogen and 20% oxygen. These molecules come from the air.

Plant roots absorb the protein and mineral content from dead bacteria in the form of white crystals, which are transferred to the leaves.

The protein immediately combines with the nitrogen from rainwater to become natural nitrogen fertilizer. The protein is also converted into amino acids by the aerobic bacteria in the leaves through the process of photosynthesis, becoming nutrients for the plants.

Rain deposits oxygen in the soil, which is essential to the roots as well as to the insects and microbes in the soil.

Dead bacteria contain organic mineral components.

Animals require Yang minerals such as sodium (Na), lithium (Li) and arsenic (As). Plants require Yin minerals such as nitrogen (N), phosphorus (P) and potassium (K). Plants suffer when they are deficient in selenium (Se), arsenic (As), phosphorus (P) and zinc (Zn), while calcium (Ca), magnesium (Mg), zinc (Zn), iodine (I) and phosphorus (P) help them grow substantially.

Plants dislike synthetic nitrogen fertilizer.

2. Comprehensive amino acids and mineral components are essential for more vigorous cell growth of larger vegetables.

Among all vegetables, *Amaranthus* from Peru contains the most amino acids. In Bolivia, it is also known as quinoa. NASA includes *Amaranthus* in its space food for its concentrated nutritional value. The amount of aspartic acid contained in *Amaranthus* is, as shown in the table below, 1.2mg/100g. Seaberry, maca and *Cordyceps militaris (Cordyceps sinensis)* contain 50 to 980mg/100g.

As for minerals, *Amaranthus* contains 152mg/100g of calcium, while butterbur and giant kelp each contain anywhere from 1600 to 2000mg/100g.

The liquid fertilizer produced by the Global Family is a fermented broth of plant bacteria that contains massive amounts of amino acids.

Vegetables will taste better if given an increased amount of amino acids.

Conventional agriculture neglects these facts because it ignores the importance of amino acids, and feeds soil only with inorganic nitrogen, phosphorus and potassium.

Plants with the most amino acids (mg/100g)

	Amaranthus (Highest among all vegetables)	Fu tea	Seaberry	Maca	Zhenjiang Vinegar concentrated	*Cordyceps militaris* (Cordyceps sinensis)	Moringa	Bidens (Beggarticks)
Lysine	0.86	7.8	68	54.5	120	980	661	—
Phenylalanine	0.62	7.5	51	55.3	110	570	1257	—
Isoleucine	0.55	5.7	38	47.4	120	520	991	—
Aspartic acid	1.22	12.7	490	91.7	300	1540	2067	—

Amaranthus **(produced in Okinawa) contains the highest amount of amino acids among all vegetables**

Plants with the highest amount of minerals (mg/100g)

	Amaranthus	Fu tea	Butterbur	Maca	Giant Kelp	Moringa	Bidens (Beggarticks)
Calcium	152	74.8	1600	220	2000	3087	1800
Magnesium	?	228	400	55.3	750	512	381
Zinc	?	2.72	3.3	3.8	6.6	4.3	6.7
Iron	111	81.7	?	15.5	6.0	9.3	13.5

To use the Global Family liquid soil improver, till the soil to a level of about 15-20 cm deep, then pour it into the soil, using approximately 60 liters per one hectare.

Bacteria that normally inhabit the leaves become sterilized by pesticides and herbicides, so it is necessary to return those bacteria to the leaves.

To do so, dilute with water by 50 times the fermented broth of leaf bacteria, which contains minerals to help the rapid and improved growth of the plant, and spray the solution directly onto the leaves.

The fermented broth of leaf bacteria is made of giant kelp, butterbur, and organic zinc-rich plants such as bidens, moringa and pines.

Nutritional value of vegetables has been on the decline year over year.

	Vegetables	1950	1963	1980	2005
Vitamin C	Spinach	150	100	65	35
	Cauliflower	80	50	65	81
	Komatsuna (Japanese mustard spinach)	90	90	75	39
	Shungiku (edible mums)	50	50	21	19

Iron	Spinach	13.3	3.3	3.7	2.0
	Garlic chives	19.0	2.1	0.6	0.7
	Shungiku (edible mums)	9.0	3.5	1.0	1.7
	Green onions	17.0	1.2	0.5	0.4
Calcium	Japanese Kabocha squash	44	44	17	20
	Winter squashes	56	56	24	15
	Japanese parsley	86	86	33	34
	Chives	85	85	120	20

Japan Food Research Laboratories (mg / 100 g)

• **Vegetables are inherently medicinal.**

1) Garlic ... high in vitamin B1, antibacterial, beneficial for immune system, chest pain, toothache, nosebleed, beriberi, rheumatoid arthritis, connective tissue disease, neuralgia, blood pressure.

2) Ginger ... high in potassium, thins blood, beneficial for coughs, internal chills, sweating, diarrhea, irritations, pain, cold, sterilization, food poisoning, blood circulation.

3) Spinach ... constipation, hemorrhoids, blood circulation, functions of the five organs, better skin, blood pressure, blood glucose level.

4) Cabbage ... cleans blood, gastrointestinal conditions, prevention of cancer, hemostasis.

5) Chinese cabbage ... health of the stomach, blood purification, stress, elimination of bowel waste, constipation, anticancer, elimination of alcohol poisoning.

6) Tomato ... controls excess heat in the blood, helps with liver functions, great for gastrointestinal diseases, helps the digestion of fat.

7) Cucumber ... blood purification, tissue purification, diuresis, swelling, gastrointestinal conditions, prevention of cancer, hemostasis.

8) Garlic chives ... enhance the gastrointestinal, liver and kidney functions, strengthen hip and knee joints, strengthen reproductive functions, improve chills and blood circulation.

9) Green onion ... antipyretics by sweating, relieves joint aches from colds by sweating and improves energy flow, decreases the swelling from inflammation and detoxifies.

●**Liquid fertilizer for Chinese medicinal vegetables** has been developed. Simply dilute with water by 50 times and spray three times onto the leaves.

Effective medicinal ingredients ... germanium, selenium, saponin, vanadium and beta carotene. Fermentation broth with medicinal ingredients of cordyceps sinensis, ginseng and snow lotus.

Cure-all effects. The vegetables will help blood, meat and bone regeneration, cell metabolism, blood purification and blood flow, and heal other symptoms.

Effective for colon cancer, lung cancer, liver cancer, autism, breast cancer, kidney cancer, pneumoconiosis, stomach cancer, muscular dystrophy, brain tumor, senile dementia, hypoxia, hangover, myocardial infarction, upper laryngeal cancer, rheumatism, Hepatitis C, gout, obesity, anemia, epilepsy, atopic dermatitis, migraines, seasonal allergies, constipation, arteriosclerosis, improvement of blood, hair growth, stress reduction, menopause, menstrual cycle irregularity.

3. Combatting weeds and improving soil's ability to support re-planting are simple

The cause of weed growth has been explained. It turns out that when the minerals in soil become deficient by growing vegetables year after year, weeds that contain those particular minerals start to grow. There are fields where horsetails grow, and those where they don't. Horsetail contains a large amount of calcium, and is alkaline. When the soil becomes acidic and below pH 4, it signals the horsetail seeds that it's time to sprout. They germinate, grow, then wither and fall to the ground to neutralize the soil with the alkaline calcium they contain. When the pH in the soil rises to levels closer to neutral (4 or above) the horsetail seeds are signaled that it is no longer their turn to grow, so they will not germinate.

The weeds that grow on the same land vary year by year. That is because those that grow are always the ones that contain the minerals lacking in the soil. There are many types of weeds that grow in farm fields; as many as the kinds of minerals there are in the soil. The ten most persistent weeds that grow in any particular field, when their effects are combined, will cover all the nutritional needs of the soil from the minerals that have been deficient there.

The bacteria that live in the leaves of those weeds contribute unique mineral components, so if you mix all ten of them, they will become a completely balanced mineral liquid. The broth from fermented leaves can become a comprehensive fertilizer for the soil in that field. It is possible to produce nutrition for the soil using only the weeds that grow in the field.

Let's talk about the failure of soil to support replanting. For example, eggplants cannot be repeatedly planted on the same plot of land, because the roots of eggplants absorb all of the nutrients in the soil needed for their growth in one season.

The bacteria inhabiting eggplant leaves are unique to eggplants, producing the necessary nutrients for them. If you cultivate the bacteria from the leaves of eggplants by fermentation and return them to the soil, the soil becomes rich in the nutrients that are necessary to eggplants, so they will grow larger and more nutritious.

Ginseng cannot be grown on the same plot of land for 8 consecutive years, but, just as with eggplants, if the microorganisms of the leaves are cultivated and returned to the soil, the problem is solved. It is now possible to repeat planting.

4. Successfully developed, safe pesticides, or pest-preventive liquid!

Common pesticides are harmful to humans. On the other hand, medicinal herbs are safe. Among the herbs that are medicinal, there are those that can effectively stop the activities of insects and animals. Some of the medicines used by the Ainu (the indigenous people of northern Japan and Russia) are poisonous to foxes and crows.

Monkshood kills animals, but is medicinal to humans. The medicine is known as Fu Zi, or aconite. Animals have a sensitive sense of smell. Nicotine is a medicinal herb with a strong smell.

Healthy plant cells deter pests. As mentioned earlier, insects are on a mission to not leave behind a species that is poorly nourished and with damaged recessive genes. Healthy and nutritious vegetables, on the contrary, try to protect themselves.

The nutrition-rich growth enhancement liquid was sprayed onto the leaves of broccoli. After just a little while, five or six caterpillars fell from the leaves to the ground. As the leaves received the nutrient-rich solution, the caterpillars decided that they must not eat the broccoli since it was high in nutrients, so they fell onto the ground to move to other fields with vegetables that were malnourished.

The insect, just like the weed seeds, judges what should be preserved and what should not be able to produce seeds.

Tall plants grow in groups in swampy areas. Every year, the waterfowls build their nests in different spots, either closer to the water's edge or on higher ground away from the water.

Waterfowls predict the weather every year. In years when heavy rainfall is expected, they build their nests on higher grounds away from the water.

In Chiba prefecture, just south of Tokyo, there were people who grew maize. When the maize was ripe enough, they came to the fields to harvest, only to find that half of the crop had been eaten by racoons. However, after they sprayed animal repellent, the racoons stopped coming.

Large-scale earthquakes or tsunamis occur from time to time, but wild animals are hardly ever found dead. When tectonic plates begin to shift, they emit unusual electromagnetic waves. Animals detect these waves and move away.

5. Harmful substances in the soil can be neutralized in one month

Various harmful substances, such as pesticides and herbicides that were used in the past remain in the soil. Among them are mercury and other heavy metals, radioactive materials, sodium and oils.

According to the principle of light energy generation, two circles of light are rotating at the speed of 1.86 trillion rotations per second. This rapid rotation fuses the atoms and electrons, and at the same time increases the number of electrons. Since increasing the number of electrons in dioxin will convert it into a different substance, this principle changes its nature and makes it become non-toxic. An increased number of electrons in cesium will cause it to no longer be cesium, making the element non-radioactive.

Bacteria supply oxygen by photosynthesis. Since oxygen itself is a form of energy, it is always light and gas at the same time. Oxygen detoxifies radioactivity.

Harmful substances lose their toxicity when placed under a controlled neutral environment.

When a patient is told by a doctor that he or she has one week to live, if you neutralize 70 to 80 percent of his or her bodily fluid, the symptoms will cease.

Radiation is highly acidic. Washing radiation-exposed clothing with strongly alkaline water neutralizes the clothing and makes it harmless.

Acidic pesticides adhere to vegetables. Dipping the vegetables in strongly alkaline water of pH 11 for one minute will neutralize them. The vegetables will taste great, just as they used to taste a long time ago.

There is such a thing as ionized calcium powder. Adding just a smidgen of it to two liters of water makes the water strongly alkaline with a pH of 11. Soaking vegetables and fruits that were sprayed with pesticides in this solution for one to two minutes will neutralize the acidity of the pesticides and render them harmless, so they will taste like they were originally intended to in the past.

Contemporary science is ignoring the laws of nature by creating synthetic chemicals and substances with molecular structures that have been disrupted and manipulated.

Nature constitutes the fusion of two elements; atoms (oxygen, +)

and electrons (hydrogen, –). People do not realize that all substances made by artificially separating and disassembling these elements have side effects.

Fusion and integration can be expressed as this: $1 + 1 = 1 \pm 0$ (neutral). The world is "oxygen + hydrogen = substance."

Modern science has ignored the providence of the natural world. It has destroyed nature and destroyed the health of living things, leading to the extinction of plant and animal species. The damage is irreversible because the majority of us do not understand the true cause of the destruction. It is not cancer, nor viral diseases.

We do not understand that the physics and chemistry targeting the missing elements is fake. The law that works for oxygen and hydrogen is what I refer to as God. It is realistic, and is the essence of science itself.

The Creator created the natural world. The Creator is the almighty wise one. He only creates things that are perfect. He creates the laws of the universe that govern all of the universe and nature, and manages the execution of these laws. The natural world is the blessing of heaven that is given to mankind, but modern science does not understand it.

The 21st century is the dawn of the era of understanding the laws of the universe and nature, applying and reproducing them.

A society in which all religions, academic disciplines and philosophies are unified by the laws of the universe is coming soon. When everything is unified, there will be no fighting. The absolute truth and the eternal law will be understood and practiced in another four to five years.

The realization of the Utopian society is near. In the Bible it is predicted that the time will come when God will be unveiled to all, when the heavenly door will be opened.

6. Viral diseases are prevalent in agriculture, livestock, and human society

Humans view bacteria as bad germs and kill them. Those who kill are killed ... A counterattack by the viruses and bacteria upon mankind has begun.

There are a lot of catastrophic viruses occurring where nature has been destroyed, or in a society focused on money, material goods and selfish concerns.

Viral diseases are also occurring in the agricultural world, but that often is not being understood, and therefore neglected.

Silver leaf disease is spreading among tomato growers' greenhouses throughout Japan. This is caused by lice, but the virus introduced through them comes at a later stage. Currently there is no countermeasure for them. The leaves of papaya turn pale, and prevent the fruits from forming. In the Philippines, a banana rotting disease has started and is spreading to southeast Asia. Livestock-oriented influenza is occurring everywhere.

In Japan, also, viral diseases are prevalent in humans. These kinds of diseases are spreading on a global scale. Modern medicine does not understand the cause nor the extent of the disease, so the administrative agencies of governments fall silent. But there exist in nature the means to sterilize viruses.

Notable remedies are propolis, which is made in the hives of honeybees, and plants such as shell ginger. They can eliminate the hepatitis C virus as well as the influenza virus in henhouses.

Silver leaf disease, which occurs in tomatoes, has also been cured. The illness affecting the bananas in the Philippines has also been suppressed by using the fermented broth that the Global Family has created.

Nature has a solution for each and every problem.

Nature is not to be overcome, but we are to coexist with it in symbiosis and to integrate ourselves with it. The Western way of thinking is focused on conflict, struggle, and human-centric concerns.

The way of living in the 21st century is to be in harmony with nature.

Currently, there is no treatment against a viral disease known as SARS (Severe Acute Respiratory Syndrome). However, when a SARS patient is orally administered the herbal fermented broth, they are cured. This is because the bacteria within the fermented broth communicate with the virus within the SARS patient. "This liquid is made by the friends of bacteria," it says. The SARS virus, understanding it, then replies, "Okay, then we will stop releasing the viral toxins."

7. Solutions to various problems in agriculture

Although modern agriculture is laden with problems, their causes have been elucidated, so it is now possible to solve various problems.

Here is an introduction to the types and the usages of the fermented broth developed for agriculture.

Types and usages of agricultural fermented broth
  (1) Integrated Liquid Soil Improver: 60 liters per 100 m²
  (2) Weed control liquid: 30 liters per 100 m²
      ① Universal type
      ② Individual type ... developed from the weeds in the particular field it will be applied to
  (3) Leaf spray (promotes growth): dilute with water by 50 to 100 times and apply directly onto the leaves. (Apply only 1 to 3

times during the life of the plant or limit to once a week)

(4) Water vitalization liquid: inject into 2 to 4 liters of water per 100 m^2

(5) Pest control solution: Dilute with water by 200 to 300 times and spray onto leaves and on the soil.

(6) Viral disease preventive solution: Dilute with water by 200 to 300 times and spray onto leaves and on the soil.

(7) Animal deterrent: Sprinkle on leaves and soil diluted with 100-300 times water

(8) Fermented broth for Chinese medicinal vegetables (Ge, Se, Li, Zn, P, Sa): Dilute with water by 50 to 100 times and spray directly onto leaves.

(9) For beta carotene (astaxanthin): Dilute by 50 to 100 times and apply onto leaves.

(10) Mending soil that has been too damaged for replanting: apply 30 liters of undiluted solution to the soil.

(11) Radioactivity decontamination: apply just enough to moisten the leaves and soil.

(12) Liquid for the breakdown of toxins in the soil: to break down mercury, dioxin, pesticide, radioactive materials, sodium, oil, heavy metal etc. Dosage varies depending on the land size. Please consult with us.

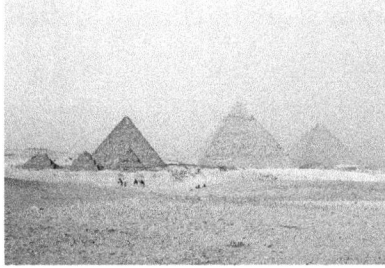

CHAPTER FIVE

Innovation in the livestock industry

1. Livestock businesses are in chronic deficit, but can be immediately improved

Most livestock feed is imported from other countries. The prices rely on overseas prices; there are no pricing rights on the Japanese side. Since the price of meat is determined by international prices, the voices and conditions on the Japanese side are not reflected.

As a result, the livestock industry is in a state of chronic deficit.

Livestock feed costs approximately 500 to 800 USD per ton. The only countermeasure to lower costs in the industry is to lower the cost of feed.

Cows only digest about half of the grass they eat, and the rest passes into their manure.

Pigs and chickens' manure contains two-thirds of undigested feed. Fermenting the manure once over will create fermented feed with the highest level of nutrients.

The leaves of sweet potato and soy are not used. Tofu (bean curd) refuse is considered industrial waste. Fermenting these food items would turn them into most nutritious feed. Only the seed parts of corn and soybeans are used. Fermenting the leaves and stems of them, and at the same time using the undiluted multi-amino acids and the multi-minerals, will turn them into feed with a complete nutrition profile.

Even better, this most nutritious livestock feed can be created within two hours of processing.

By this method, the cost of feed, which is currently around six hundred dollars per ton will be reduced significantly to about 50 to 60 dollars, while giving the livestock the best nutrients ever. All livestock will immediately eat it.

So far, the completely fermented manure has been preferred by cows, pigs and chickens. Goldfish in ponds and cats eat this as well.

This feed, when fermented with the undiluted multi-amino acids and the multi-minerals, becomes a feed with comprehensive nutrients, and deodorizes the livestock excreta.

Mr. T, a farmer in Obihiro, in the northern island of Hokkaido, who raises 140 milking cows, had requested the fermented broth. He mixed 1 liter of fermented broth in a 1000-liter water tank and gave it to his cows. After two weeks of administering this water, his veterinarian came to visit the barn. The vet told him that the barn did not have the bad odor that it did before.

One of his cows developed a condition that is equivalent to cancer in humans.

Mr. T gave the fermented broth to the sick cow to drink. Then the cow was healed. The veterinarian told him that he had been caring for animals for 28 years and it was the first time he had seen a cow with this kind of illness be cured.

In Kumamoto in southern Japan also, cattle with pneumonia or leukemia were healed.

When I entered the barn in Obihiro, I spoke to two cows. Without making sounds, I talked to them in my mind. I said to them that their lives and my life were equally precious, then smiled at them.

The cows glanced at me and acted as if nothing happened.

The farmer told me that, when strangers enter his barn, the cows usually become restless. He wondered how they kept calm on that day.

You see, all lives are equal, so we can speak to one another.

In Okinawa, the southernmost island of Japan, I entered a barn with 150 pigs, and sprayed their noses with the fermented broth that was developed as a skin care product for humans. Far from having animosity, about 20 pigs came rushing toward me and begged me to spray them.

The pigs recognized that this was medicinal. As I left the barn, all 150 pigs started squealing loudly, wanting to be sprayed. Immediately, the owner of the pigs asked me for the formula of the fermented broth.

The characteristics of livestock drinking water (with fermented broth) - It is made from medicinal herbs that are equal or more effective than they are for human beings.

· For better cell growth, herbs that contain bacteria on the plants that are rich in organic zinc - Giant kelp, bidens, butterbur. Herbs with multi-amino acids - Moringa, bidens, caterpiller fungus.
· Sterilizing viruses - shell ginger, propolis
· Better digestion of feed - bacteria that break down grass in the gastric juice of cattle help reduce the energy necessary for digestion.
· The best Himalayan medicinal herbs to promote cures for incurable diseases - Snow lotus, Tibet ginseng
· Ataractic for stress relief - herbs from Andean mountains, Himalayas, India, and other Chinese medicinal herbs

2. The effect of the fermented broth using the above herbs:

Deodorizing livestock excreta, treatment of diseases, stress relief, growth promotion, improved quality of meat, enhanced digestive ability ·· energy used for digestion is now channeled to the production of meat and milk.

Livestock know that humans consume their meats.

Therefore, they must be raised with plenty of love and care. When the stalls are kept smelly and unsanitary, it causes stress on the animals. Their eyes become dull and hateful instead of being clear. Their health can be measured by how clear or unclear their eyes are.

It is possible to increase the amount of DHA and beta carotene contained within chicken eggs.

Because both components act as antioxidants, these eggs will not expire for about six months.

Consumption of these eggs will result in higher brain capacity and healing of all diseases.

DHA is mostly contained in mackerel, sardines, and squid innards. Fermenting these is known to increase the DHA by three times.

Haematococcus pluvialis (Microalgae) produces astaxanthin, which becomes beta carotene, and turns red. Giving this fermented broth to chickens will turn the eggshells a brighter red. The eggs can be sold for 100 yen (about one dollar) a piece.

Pigs and cows are born with hooves. Having hooves means they are 100% herbivores. They are designed to walk on soft surfaces such as soil and grass. But humans build barns with concrete floors. The stimulation from walking on concrete goes to the brain, and the stress causes them to have diarrhea. Their growth is stunted by this loss of energy. Cover the floor with hay and straw. Spraying them with the fermented broth made with microorganisms that promote oxygen production will prevent decomposition and odor.

Cattle, when raised in vast ranches, tend to walk around too much and not gain weight because the energy for growth is spent elsewhere. They prefer being raised in varied terrain, compared to flat lands.

It is necessary to make them exercise moderately, but too much exercise will result in weight loss.

The American way of running the livestock business puts too much stress on the cattle. The quality and the taste of the meat declines.

Livestock feel tremendous fear when being slaughtered. Toxins are released into their blood stream. Once, I talked to Mr. Sano, the president of a top ramen shop. I said, "I know you make the best-tasting noodles, but that pork you keep in the refrigerator is of poor quality. Put this device in the refrigerator and see what happens," and I handed him my light energy generator.

Mr. Sano later sent me a message stating that the taste of the soup he made with the pork had improved. Light energy neutralizes toxins to make them harmless, so the soup has improved.

There are children who are allergic to eggs. Placing eggs on the light energy generator for several minutes will neutralize the allergenic substances. The eggs, when consumed, will not cause any allergic reactions.

The device improves the quality and taste of meats as well.

The industry of the 21st century is a nurturing one. Vegetables, domestic animals, fish and forests all are living things.

Chiba prefecture, just south of Tokyo, investigated the condition of their forests and determined that 80% of the tree roots were decaying. Acid rain caused excessive acidity in the soil, which pushed out oxygen, so the roots started to rot.

Hydrogen water is now becoming more popular. Excessive hydrogen would spoil blood within our body.

Since modern science mainly focuses on physics and chemistry, and is centered around materials, it does not help us understand that oxygen is energy, and mass comes from hydrogen. Oxygen is the life-sustaining energy itself, and always exists as both light and gas. It is invisible.

Oxygen is the same as light, or the rays of the Sun. In Japanese we say "Okagesamade (thank heavens)." The 'sama (heavens)' implies the Sun.

The present generation does not understand this fact.

The Sun activates the atoms of the body, while the Moon, the electrons.

Nocturnal people's faces appear pale. The atom is life.

The theory that reactive oxygen causes cancer is a serious error. This way of thinking has terribly derailed the medicine.

The Sun, the Moon and the Earth are in a trinity. This trinity maintains the balance of light energy and magnetic energy between these celestial bodies, and their motions and rotations. The Sun affects the nerves, and the Moon does the menstrual cycle. The Sun governs life, while the Moon, the physiology of the body. It is all about circulation, which causes the rotation of the Earth.

Life is born at the full moon and ends at the new moon. It is the Moon that controls the physical bodies, and the Sun, life.

Without using the lunar calendar, agriculture and fishery can not be successful. But the Japanese Agricultural Cooperatives does not recommend farmers depend on such calendar.

In the fishery industry, it used to be common knowledge among fishermen that fish showed the strongest appetite at the full moon and the new moon, as well as the specific locations where the tides would flow.

Ohma in Aomori prefecture, in northern Japan, is famous for their tuna fishery. Currently the fishermen wander around the water using radars on their boats. The older generation used to know exactly how the tide flowed, and would be able to make a straight line to the best fishing ground.

The present generation has forgotten the laws of nature. Humans cannot overcome nature. The time is now to realize that fact.

The Entrances to Shambhala Around the World
The Seven Holy Sites of the World

Shambhala Headquarters

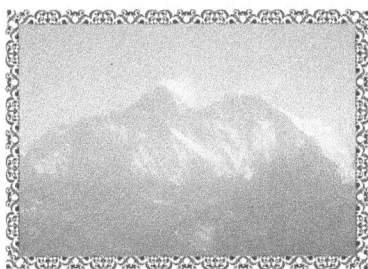

Lhotse in the Himalayas

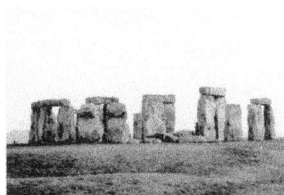

Stonehenge,
near London, UK

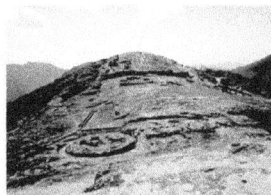

Samaipata,
Bolivia

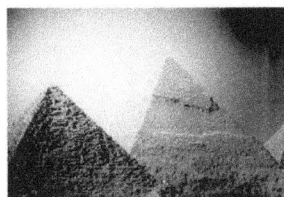

The view of the world from
the North Pole

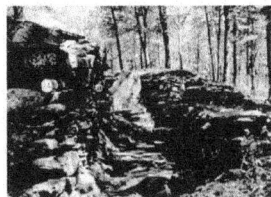

Great Pyramid of Giza

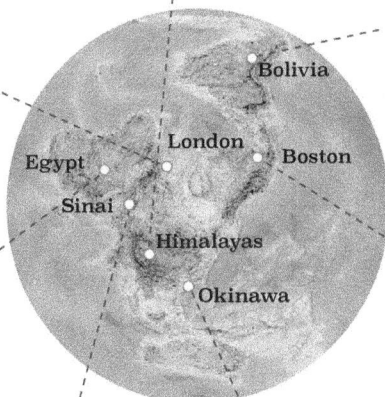

Stonehenge, near Boston
Massachusetts, USA

Mount Serbal, Sinai where
Moses is believed to have prayed

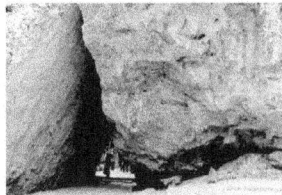

Sefa Utaki,
Okinawa, Japan

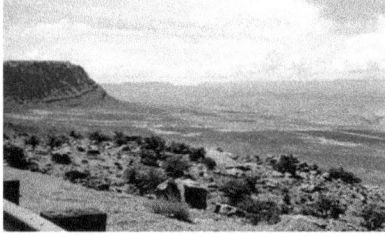

CHAPTER SIX

Divine healing of mind and body

1. Revelation of the mystery of humans and the human body

(1) The mystery of birth

Why are humans born? - this is a mystery that has not been explained. The Creator creates all things, and dwells within them as atoms and electrons. Humans were created and trained by the Creator to be the lords of all creations at the highest point of evolution. The commonly held theory of evolution is wrong. Monkeys are created as monkeys, totally separate from the creation of humans.

The Creator tells us (directly through Mr. Yoshihiko Uezu in the year 2015), "You are now born in the era of killing and deceiving. For over a thousand years, I have forged every single one of you through life experiences and reincarnations to be the leader of the Guiding Spirits. For the last five hundred years, especially, I raised you to be able to rectify these turbulent times.

Every one of you were born with the goal of promoting life, and the capability to have a role in fixing this turbulent world, and to strive for the betterment of the world and of each other. But you have forgotten about it. Wake up."

Being born as a human being in this world depends solely on the judgment of the Creator. If mere sexual intercourse would lead to conception, the Earth would have been packed with humans a long time ago.

Let me reveal to you the process of the birth of humans.

The Creator tells the soul (discarnate entity) of a person, "Manifest in a human body, be born on the earthly world and improve your soul."

The soul of the person then says, "Okay," and chooses how to eradicate its karma from the previous life, how to be trained, who should be its allies and what their roles should be. It also chooses the challengers who will sabotage it, the helpers, the teachers, etc., and even chooses his/her own parents. Finally, he/she decides on life expectancy. And all the stakeholders gather to approve what role they are to play in the discarnate entity.

When we are born, our old memories are erased upon passing through the birth canal. In the other world, there are as many as 60 billion souls waiting for their turn to be born as a human being. Within one of the sperm of any father-to-be, according to the soul's choice, the Creator plants an archeocell (Cosmos cell), which contains the complete genetic structure of the Creator.

This cell is infused with the almighty wisdom. It creates blood, muscles and bones to give a unique functionality to each of the other cells within, to make up a whole and complete body. Only the sperm that contains this Cosmos cell will be able to bind with the mother-to-be's egg and move forward to conception.

As soon as the egg is fertilized, the process of cell division begins. The baby is then nurtured for nine months in the amniotic fluid to become a complete human form, until it is time for birth.

The fetus does not breathe air. It is not alive yet.

Nutrients and oxygen are received through the umbilical cord. There are two cords that keep humans alive. The Cosmos cell is the source of the Creator's cosmic life. It is also considered as another umbilical cord.

Life is sustained through those two umbilical cords.

The soul is a living organism given by the Creator. It is the Creator's alter ego, its spirit and soul. Each soul has a unique personality, according to the various experiences from its previous life.

Each soul is destined to eventually unite with the cosmic life of the Creator. Like it or not, it has to be done.

At the moment the baby is released from the amniotic fluid, his/her soul enters the body and gives its first cry. The birthing process is then complete. If there were no cry, the baby would be stillborn. Memorial services would be held. Death occurs when a soul is released before it has entered the physical body.

After birth, the Cosmos cell settles inside the heart, leading the bacteria to transform the food that the person consumes into blood, muscle, bones and cells. It keeps working nonstop, 24-hours a day to make sure that all the systems function according to their unique roles.

During pregnancy, the physical body of a baby is created through the unification of a sperm (oxygen, atom) and an egg (hydrogen, electron). The soul that is going to occupy the baby stays close to the mother until childbirth. The mother is able to communicate with the discarnate entity that will be the soul of the baby. Birth is science, but it also has mystical elements. Therefore, women who have experienced childbirth tend to have stronger psychic abilities than men.

Mothers would say that they gave birth to their babies. However, human beings are not capable of creating a single drop of blood nor an organ. Babies have the ability to communicate with discarnate entities. Children of the 21st century live in an evolving era, therefore they are more evolved than their parents. Children up to the age of 12 can communicate with spirits. But adults do not understand this fact, which makes the children feel distrustful towards them, thinking that the adults know nothing.

(2) Human behavior

Breathing

People do not understand exactly why we breathe. It is to inhale the life energy known as oxygen in the air. We die within three minutes of not breathing.

The oxygen level in the air is 20.9%. A level of less than 19 to 18% would cause altitude sickness. Less than 18 to 17% could cause brain death, which we often hear about as a cause of accidental death in manholes and holding tanks. There is no pain or suffering associated with brain death. Such is the case with death by hanging.

Corpses decompose because there is no breath to inhale oxygen.

We are all kept alive by oxygen, an invisible substance. Furthermore, the exhaled breath contains the unfiltered thought waves of a person. They vary between short-tempered and patient people.

In the Japanese language, the character for the word "breathe" is a combination of "self" and "heart." There is a breathing technique known as Prāṇāyāma.

There is a slight increase in the population when people live on less food intake.

When we practice Prāṇāyāma, we consciously inhale the life energy (oxygen) within the air. This way, we can take in far more energy than through merely breathing without being mindful.

When we completely exhale all the air from our lungs, inhalation becomes nice and smooth. Many people emit destructive energy in their exhaled breath. The exhalations of money-, material- and self-obsessed people are full of destructive vibrations, which accumulate in the tectonic plates and eventually cause earthquakes.

China is in danger. The minimum oxygen concentration in people's blood is said to be around 12 ppm. When the temperature rises by 1 degree Celsius, the oxygen concentration decreases by 1 ppm.

In humans, an increase of 3 ppm will cause brain death. Whales sometimes wash up on the shore because they become brain dead near the shore.

The coral reefs in the ocean are dying because the temperature of the sea water is rising, lowering the oxygen concentration in the water. The water is literally dead. No creature would be able to sustain life in such a place.

(3) The balance of energy within the human body

The rotary motion of energy always flows in a whirl, either sinistral or dextral. Through this, the universe and human beings keep their balance.

Sinistral → absorb ... low pressure in atmosphere, left brain
---reception, left eye and ear
Dextral → emit ... high pressure in atmosphere, right brain
---transmission, right eye and ear

The brain can only function or 'rotate' when a balance of ins and outs is achieved. E-mail is only for "in." People tend to steer away from phone calls and start being dependent on e-mails, which keep stuffing the INboxes. There is only INput, just catching data, and this system is lacking outlets or ways of expression - causing people to become stubborn and hardened. Now, those people, without exception, develop stiffness in the left-side of their body - knots in their shoulder, back pain, and/or leg pain. They might even have headache, migraines, psychotic disorders, or paralysis. E-mails are a one-way communication, without the circulation of ins and outs. The energy flow becomes abnormal. It is similar to energy paths in the nervous system. In the Japanese language, the combination of the characters for "God" and "paths" form the word for "nerves."

Functions of the body

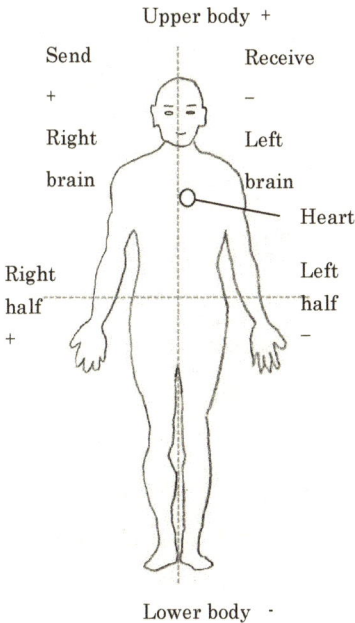

Upper body +

Send   Receive

+   −

Right   Left

brain   brain

           Heart

Right   Left

half   half

+   −

Lower body ·

o Human body is divided in terms of Yin and Yang parts to circulate the energy flow. >>> IN-OUT ion exchanges.

o Upper body is + (Yang), lower body is − (Yin). The spiritual realm is +, Material realm is −.

>>>People of the material realm have elongated lower bodies and longer legs.

o Left hand is − and is for absorption. Right hand is + and is for emission. Energy circulates from the right to left hand.

· i.e. Hands on the statues of Buddha and Jizo Bodhisattva have the right hand (emission) up for giving things to people. They hold the left hands (absorption) up to receive things from people.

· Throughout the world, we put both hands together to pray.

· The median of + and − is neutral. God, as well as nature, is neutral.

oLight (waves) emitted from the right eye.

· The light bounces off an object and is caught by the left eye.

oSound waves (vibrations) emitted from the right ear.

The left ear absorbs the vibrations >>> able to sense the distance

oIN through the mouth, OUT through the anus >>> circulation.

·Schools tend to cram children's brains. In modern society, children are bound by the disciplines of the organizations they belong to. At home, they live in constraints, without any place to express their true feelings. They could develop any type of malady, from headache, to minor depression and neurosis, to autism, severe depression or psychosis. They only need to be given the opportunity and the space to diversify their feelings. Remember, the brain will not function or ‹rotate› until the balance of ins and outs is achieved.

· Generation of energy

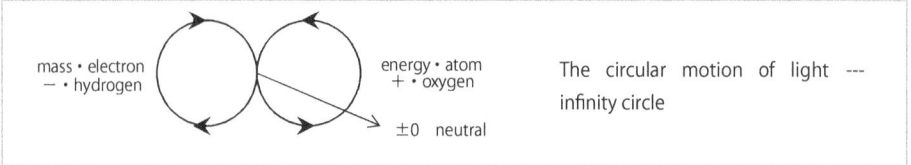

mass · electron
— · hydrogen

energy · atom
+ · oxygen
±0   neutral

The circular motion of light ---
infinity circle

Energy is generated through the balance of light, oxygen and hydrogen. The maximum speed of the two rotational movements within light is 1.86 trillion times per second. This rotation causes the oscillation, or vibration of energy. This rotation produces frictional heat within cells, to achieve the normal body temperature of 36.5 degrees Celsius.

By means of this rotation, atoms and electrons are coupled to-gether, and at the same time, as the number of electrons is increased, various elements are created.

Within our body, new blood, muscle and bones are created every three minutes, by means of elemental transmutation at room temperature.

Intolerance to cold is caused by the lower level of oxygen in the body slowing down the rotation of light, or energy, which in turn decreases the frictional heat within the body. When the ability for elemental transmutation weakens, it becomes more difficult for the body to make new blood, muscle and bones. This is the cause of in-fertility. The two rotational movements mentioned above are what I call "Hyotan kara Koma," meaning something very unexpected can come out of something ordinary.

· **Cells function like batteries. They generate energy.**

Cell membrane

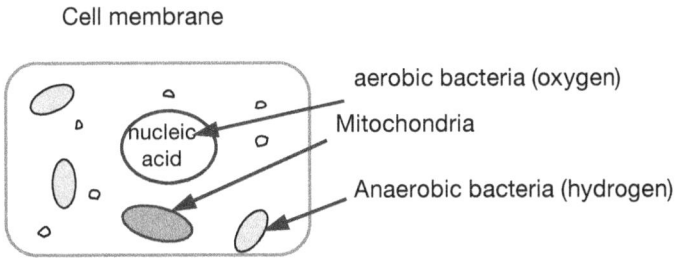

aerobic bacteria (oxygen)

nucleic acid

Mitochondria

Anaerobic bacteria (hydrogen)

Cells are battery devices that generate light energy by means of oxygen and hydrogen. The energy is then used for cell division. When the balance of energy is lost, cells die. By utilizing this energy, cells can keep renewing and rejuvenating the body through the process of cell division.

Muscle cells are completely renewed every three months, while those of the bones, every five- to six-months.

People of the present generation live with an excessive amount of acid in the body.

Acidity means that the oxygen levels have been forcibly decreased. When oxygen decreases, the amount of hydrogen in the blood increases, spoiling the blood and causing all kinds of diseases. It weakens the battery function of the cells, causing decreased ability for them to divide. As the dead cells start accumulating in the body, it starts to rot, causing cancers and atopic dermatitis. When the battery function of the cells weakens, the ability to produce new blood, muscle and bones decreases, therefore the body's natural healing power decreases as well.

(4) The role of the blood

Blood supplies oxygen and nutrients to tissues in the body and collects waste products. Blood is mildly alkaline. In the natural world it has the tendency to neutralize, therefore the blood attracts oxygen, which is acidic. Oxygen is life energy. It circulates in the body by itself and moves along the hydrogen. It is the power of oxygen that circulates the liquid element of the blood. Oxygen-rich blood flows more smoothly, as it is thinner blood that is easier to circulate. Thickened, dirty blood is called "o-ketsu" (clotted blood) in Chinese medicine, and is considered to be the cause of numerous diseases.

Mental stress is one of the causes of the blood thickening. Anger, anxiety and resentment generate toxins and abnormal hormones, among other negative elements. As sodium level increases, the sodium attracts fats that thicken the blood. Potassium breaks down sodium. The thickened blood can be thinned out using a frequency of 8,000 to 10,000 hertz. There are CDs available that play sounds with this frequency (Sold by Global Family). Listening to these frequencies can decrease the risk of brain hemorrhage and stroke.

Let's not forget that blood has the ability to cleanse: ① cleanse itself, ② cleanse the internal organs, and ③ discard dead cells through sweating. The average human discards 2.5 liters of water each day. Therefore, not replenishing the same amount of water will decrease the blood's cleansing ability, which will thicken the blood and cause symptoms such as gallstones or menstrual cramps. To maintain the body's cleansing system, it is important to consume at least 2.5 liters of water each day.

The total length of the blood vessels in the head alone is at a ratio of about 1:1 to the vessels throughout the rest of the body. The eyes and brain are aggregates of capillary vessels. The number of cells in them is also 1:1 compared to cells in the rest of the body. This tells you how complicated your eyes and brain are.

The blood flow in capillaries increases with more light energy.

(5) The rhythm within the human body

① Physiological rhythm

    Breathing 12   Body temperature 36   Pulse 72   Blood pressure 144

Multiples of 4:   3   9   18   36

② Brain waves and the mind

Beta wave

13 to 30 Hz   State of egoism, excited state, pulse wave

Alpha wave

8 to 13 Hz Egoism is halved, sleeping state,

                    alternate current wave

———*Omega wave*

4 to 8 Hz Peaceful, immovable state, direct current wave

-------------*Gamma wave*

0.4 to 4 Hz Cosmic conscious state, comatose

4 Hz and 8 Hz are the wavelengths that can calm the mind.

Pulsed wave

Only able to catch one-third of the light energy from the Sun

A/C wave

Only able to catch half of the light energy from the Sun

———*D/C wave*

Able to catch 100% of the light energy from the Sun

③ Composition of the human body - Brain

The brain's weight is 1/50 of the body weight.

1/5 of the blood circulates in the brain.

It controls the 5 senses: eyes, ears, nose, tongue, skin.

5 Zang 6 Fu: Refers to five Yin organs (Heart, Liver, Spleen, Lung, Kidney) and six Yang (Small Intestine, Large Intestine, Gall Bladder, Urinary Bladder, Stomach and Sānjiaō). Sānjiaō, or "triple burner" is not an organ but a Chakra. Therefore, the correct description should be 5 Zang 5 Fu.

(6) Meaning of the seven colors of the rainbow ... Sunlight

Sunlight is clear, spread by a prism into seven colors. All seven colors mixed together makes clear. These seven colors are used in expressions such as Lucky Seven, Seven Lucky Gods, and Seven Churches. The names of the Angels of Light all end with "el." Michael, Uriel, Gabriel etc. The seven colors are collectively re-ferred as El-Ranty.

Seven is the number that is associated with completion. July 7th in Japan is interpreted as a day when everything is "Done as it should be done." There are ancient symbols connected with the number seven, such as the Big Dipper, the Seven Holy Swords and Seven Candlesticks. $7 \times 7 = 49$. This also means "completion."

There are seven hormonal control centers, or chakras, within the human body, corresponding to the seven colors of sunlight.

Among those seven centers, the thyroid gland, pancreas, and ad-renal glands are the three that directly affect health. Abnormality in any of them would lead to all kinds of illnesses.

Activating the heart chakra, the throat chakra and the third eye chakra is referred to as the alignment of the soul, which relieves the body from illness. This is the state of enlightenment. When all chakras are activated, the person is now free from all diseases. The activation of all seven chakras is the enlightenment state. Buddha described it as the opening of a lotus flower. In India, it is referred to as the opening of a peacock's tail feathers.

How the chakras work

7th: Crown chakra - connection to cosmic consciousness.
This opens after all the other six chakras are activated
...... ①Purple

6th: Third eye chakra - between the eyebrows. Vision of the
past, the present and the future. Controls intuition and
inspiration...... ②Indigo

5th: Throat chakra - controls creativity, arts, feelings of fear
and anxiety. Degradation of endotoxin. Self-preservation
instinct ...... ③Blue

4th: Heart chakra - the soul inhabits the space behind the heart.
God dwells in the heart. Thinking process originates here.
Love ...... ④Green

3rd: Solar Plexus chakra - the control center for emotions and
conflicts. Hormonal control of the pancreas. Metabolism,
internal organs ..... ⑤Yellow

2nd: Sacral chakra - Tanden (abdomen), relates to material
desires and self-preservation instinct. Anger, fear, adrenal
glands, fighting spirit, blood pressure ...... ⑥Orange

1st: Root chakra - tail bone. Instinct, lust, greed for money,
reproductive glands, life force ...... ⑦Red

The person at the lower level of the psychic spectrum develops the
first chakra abnormally. Because it can only communicate with the
lower-ranking spirits, they emit a foul odor.

When all the chakras are activated, the person will emit an aura
of white light from the body.

Telepathy can be possible through the third chakra, combined with the pituitary gland as the transmitter and the pineal gland at the crown chakra as the receiver. Understanding others without speaking and communication with the ultra-high discarnate entities are possible.

The alignment of the chakras gives people around the world this aura, and improves people's consciousness and health. It provides the best service.

The connection between the cosmic consciousness and the body is in the pineal gland. The center of the pineal gland is the center of the subconsciousness.

People are supposed to receive light energy from the crown. However, our bodies are tilted and not standing straight, making it difficult for the energy to enter properly.

When energy comes in, it flows through the spine and activate the chakras. Most people are deficient in this light energy.

Well-trained therapists are able to condition their patients' chakras so that the energy can easily enter from the crown. However, most people pay too much attention to their body, ignoring the invisible energy.

Cosmic Energy

① pineal

Pituitary gland

② cerebellum

Thyroid
③ Parathyroid

④ Heart
(thymic gland)

Liver   Stomach

⑤ pancreas

adrenal gland
kidney

⑥

⑦

Cosmic Energy

↓

pineal gland (nectar)

↑   ↓

pituitary gland

↑   Thyroid
                     (Thyroxin)

Parathyroid
(acetylcholine)

↑   ↓

Heart (thymic gland)

↑

Pancreas (insulin)

↑   ↓

                     Adrenal gland
                     (estrogen)

Kidney (adrenalin)

↑   ↓

Tailbone (gonad)

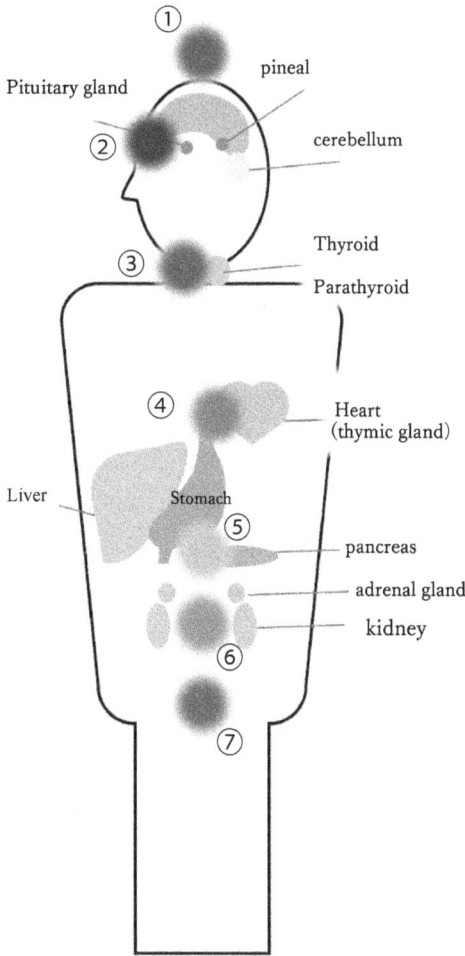

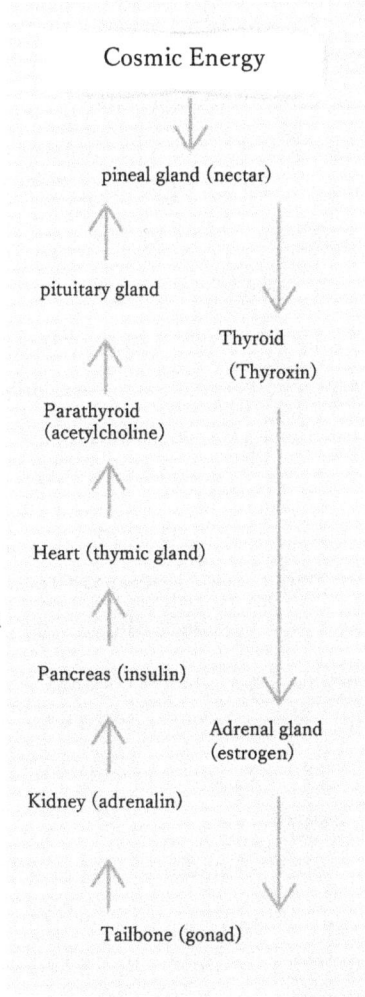

Cosmic energy circulates through the seven chakras. When one or more chakras are not active, the body will lack the life energy, causing all sorts of illnesses.

The Trinity within the human being

The human being consists of the Trinity of the body, the soul and the spiritual body. Correspondingly, there are three discarnate entities within as well. Under normal circumstances, only the consciousness is active, and as long as it is working, the remaining two, subconsciousness and superconsciousness, cannot work. This is why the shamans in Central America and Brazil eat certain types of cactus called Peyote or San Pedro, which puts the consciousness to sleep.

Information from the superconsciousness is given in a visual form. The pictures drawn by shamans who are given accurate information are very precise, because they are given this visual information. The scholars who are unaware of this fact would say that the shamans' experiences are merely hallucinations.

Meditation is one way to deactivate the consciousness. Self-guided meditation is dangerous, because a gap could be created in the mind, where the lower discarnate entities could wreak havoc. Most guidebooks on meditation available, unfortunately, do not touch upon this fact.

Meditation is about concentrating on infinite light energy, or life energy.

Superconsciousness is a Cosmos cell within our hearts. It is the cell that contains the 100%-complete genes of the Creator. The ideal meditation is to totally concentrate on this cell. All life consists of this infinite cosmic life. It is almighty. Enlightenment means to fully realize and understand that we are kept alive by this infinite cosmic life.

See, it's that simple.

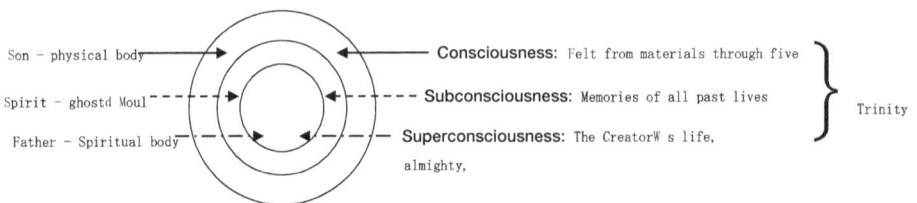

Son – physical body — Consciousness: Felt from materials through five

Spirit – ghostd Moul — Subconsciousness: Memories of all past lives

Father – Spiritual body — Superconsciousness: The CreatorW s life, almighty,

Trinity

In the Chinese language, the character for "medicine" has changed from 靈 to 醫 to 医. This hints at the progress of the field of medicine. Modern medicine does not even know what causes cancers. The only treatments available involve either removing an illness through an operation or blast radiation, or searing it with a laser. Where there is no understanding of the root cause of the illness, there are only symptomatic treatments that can relieve it. Doctors do not fully comprehend how the blood, muscle and bones are made, and who makes them.

Medicine will return to its origin

· The transition of the Chinese character for «medicine» correlates to how it is interpreted, and its approach to the natural world.

· The character for «medicine» has changed from 靈 to 醫 to 医.

Transformation of Medicine	靈	醫	医
Works of the spirits	Releasing the mind from the body Releasing into the cosmic consciousness	Balancing the body and mind (soul)	Cleansing and activating the body, improving metabolism
Shennong Bencaojing (Classic herbal medicine)	"Noble" or "upper" herbs, nourishing life, leading us closer to God and enlightened states	"Common" or "middle" herbs, nourishing bodies, prevent illness and strengthen bodies	"Low" herbs, treatments to recover from illnesses. Have side effects
Components of body and consciousness	Superconsciousness, spiritual body	Subconsciousness, soul	Consciousness, physical body

In 21st Century, medicine will return to "靈" -- and utilize the almighty wisdom to realize the Trinity.

Treatments	Communication with the consciousness, medicinal herbs, target the body and soul holistically	Medicinal herbs, fermentation, intervascular, target live physical bodies	Medicating and operating, will stall cell activities and lower immunity, target only the physical body
Therapists	Shamans, communication between heaven and earth	Therapists, target the body and soul holistically	Medical specialists, segmentation of the body into specialized areas, not able to see the big picture

2. Cause of illnesses

(1) The causes of illness are the unseen things

① Wasting money causes excess aging. Ill thoughts lead to wasted energy that is needed for the metabolism of cells, which causes the phenomenon of metabolism to not be performed well, leading to excess aging. If the body constantly metabolizes, there is aging going on. Cells are triangularly shaped, and are combined with others to form various organs. God works in scientific ways.

Wasting of a man's sperm or a women's fluid will cause the loss of metabolic energy in the cells, causing aging. This is because the energy needed for blood circulation and cell metabolism is deprived.

Having too much sexual intercourse is a waste of sperm, as well as the vaginal fluid that rejuvenates female hormones. This, again, is a waste of male and female hormones that control the blood circulation and cell metabolism. People who suppress the excretion of sperm or vaginal fluid stay younger and healthier. Old people who have little sperm or vaginal fluid left are slow to recover from injuries or illnesses. Their metabolism is not taking place efficiently, causing excess aging.

Athletes and Sumo wrestlers become weaker when they get married. Small seeping of sperm is just a release of excess and is not a problem. However, forcible release is abnormal and an excess.

② Mental state can destroy cells

Money-, material- and self-centered people tend to clash and be in continuous conflict. In those cases, the stress of the mind turns into physical illness. The vibrational frequency of argumentative people is geared to destruction. Their cells are rough and emit a ravaging frequency. Some of those cells leave the organs they belong to, and wander alone to rot. These become cancer cells.

Some cells decide to behave selfishly, they begin to eat the adjacent cells and start growing. These are also cancer cells. Cosmos cells exist behind the heart. The Cosmos cells produce sperm. The more exquisite the mind is, the more exquisite the cells are. The number of cells would then increase. When the cells become ethereal, one will be able to have out-of-body experiences. This is because the cells become smaller and more transparent.

The Cosmos cells change normal cells from being particles to becoming elementary particles. They create other cells with the same triangular shape. When lacking love, cells divide abnormally to become cells with destructive thoughts. With love, the number of cells with love will increase, emitting the vibrational frequency of love. Without love, cells will separate and repulse other cells, destroying the cells and the whole body.

Feelings of anger and hatred especially have an enormous power of destruction. These feelings literally annihilate the body from within. Too many cells die this way. Destruction of such scale leads to parts of the body being unable to sustain cells. This is also the birth of cancer cells. When the mind is in harmony, cancer never occurs. When the mind is filled with love and harmony, the body has the power of attraction, and can communicate within to produce stronger affinity. The cells will never rot or wander to become cancerous. When a person holds onto a sense of separation and feels as though other people are different from themselves, the cells start separating and wandering.

The number of cells in the body differs from person to person. Loving and harmonious people have as many as 70 to 80 trillion cells that can become ethereal and light. Cosmos cells divide the cell particles into finer particles and keep the body healthy. Ill-minded people's cells contain many dead or blackened cells, which cause all sorts of illnesses. Cancer cells are not alive, and not functional. Anger and hatred generated by a person keep destroying their own cells, causing cancer to spread.

③ The cause of sick cells – "as the mind thinketh"
Most people believe that they are human beings who are different from others. This thought of differentiation leads to conflict, causing the mental stress which in turn becomes physical illness.

When there is a sense of conflict in our thoughts, a chemical reaction occurs in our cells. The cells separate, as the thoughts intended. The cells then are in conflict with and separate from each other, and start rotting. Short-tempered people are angry. A short-temper causes cell destruction within the body and damages many cells, causing them to die.

Every time you lose your temper, many more cells die. Toxins form spontaneously, which enter the blood stream to circulate around the body. A type of toxin forms and causes various kinds of damage within the body. This toxin can kill many cells, accelerating the aging process. It also causes illness.

The entire time you spend hating others, your cells are also repelling, destroying and killing each other. You must understand this as fact.

When you love someone, your cells attract each other and become healthy. We must understand that suicidal thoughts are a form of illness that have deep roots within a person.

We should also know that the Cosmos cell itself, which derives from the Creator, will never become ill. Only the cells that are created by the Cosmos cells can be destroyed. Our physical body is controlled by the Cosmos cells. Whether we become healthy or sick really depends on our state of mind.

④ Feelings like resentment, fear and anger emit vibrational frequencies that can take over the cells. Typical cells live for three months. In that duration, the cells can, without the intention of the mind, emit vibrational frequencies of anger and fear. This is why it is so important to control your mind.

Most people only believe in what they see, and rarely turn their attention to the unseen things. If the causes of illness are unseen factors, shouldn't we consider healing those for the cures to our illnesses?

Our bodies, which are visible, are collections of atoms and electrons, all of which are invisible to the naked eye. Thus, the unseen is the cause, as well as the result. The present generation ignores the world of causes, which consists of atoms and electrons. They are blind and ignorant, living within a closed body. The only way to truly know what is happening within the body is through spiritual vision. Discordant hearts create diseases. There are women who can see through their vision the specific changes in the body that take place when ingesting medicinal herbs. Saints and shamans can have this spiritual vision. When someone says that he is a good person, the spiritual sense of vision might see otherwise. This is what Jesus meant when he said that illnesses are the signs of sins.

Discordant minds, in addition to ignoring the spirit and only seeing the physical realm, are the cause of illness. When the mind is filled with love and harmony, there is no destruction within the body's cells. The state of our minds is most important. Hatred, anger, jealousy, judging others - those are the causes of disharmony within us. Our perspectives are relative. Few people have an absolutely harmonious mind.

As I mentioned before, the number of cells in the body differs from person to person. A loving person has more cells and emanates ethereal vibrational frequencies. Cosmos cells behind the heart are the very particles that control and divide cells. They keep the body healthy. Noble people and people with high energy, without exception, have a higher number of cells. Ill-minded people's bodies contain many dead or blackened cells, which cause all sorts of illnesses. Cancer cells are not alive, and not functional. The anger and hatred of a person can keep destroying their own cells, causing cancer to spread.

When a person is filled with God's love and harmony, the Cosmos cells order the body to produce more new cells. Any illness, including cancer, is cured. It is the sick person who is causing the body not to heal. Ill thoughts waste the cells' energy, preventing good metabolism. New cells fill up the gaps left by old cells, but they have no power to fill them. The present generation disregards the importance of a healthy mind.

(2) On attaining Buddhahood in one lifetime and out-of-body experiences - science as mystery

① Jesus' cross and the resurrection on the third day

Cosmos cells have the vibrational frequencies of love and harmony. The most exquisite vibrational frequency is attained when a body becomes so ethereal that it evaporates. When someone dies but does not leave a body behind, it is sometimes described as the attainment of Buddhahood. Jesus died on the cross, and returned the body to heaven. He resurrected after three days by the materialization of his physical body. He then returned to heaven at the age 69 in Kashmir, India, without leaving his body behind. This fact was written on an ancient wooden plank in a certain temple in India.

When Cosmos cells and the soul escape from the body, the body become soul-less. This is death. Jesus preached, "One must not be born again within the physical body."

Ethereal cells are invisible, yet they can appear through the phenomenon of materialization. There is no need to use mothers' wombs. This is called Mai-Lupa. On the full moon day of May every year, the Wesak Festival is held at Mount Kailash in Tibet. On this day, Buddha and Jesus appear in the physical form. People who can have out-of-body experiences have ethereal cells. Moses, Jesus, as well as Mr. Toshihiko Chibana all have had out-of-body experiences at will.

There is an old saying that not connecting with God is unfruitful. When Cosmos cells are working perfectly, the cells become more exquisite for better sensory abilities, being able to catch more information sent from the higher discarnate entities. Recognizing the reality of Cosmos cells is described as the arrival of the spirits. Because most humans emanate lower frequencies, they are not compatible with the higher frequencies of Jesus' consciousness, thus they cannot see Him.

Leave everything to Cosmos cells. By letting everything go, your vibrational frequency becomes higher, your body and mind lighter, and you become able to enter the so-called private place. We say, "Pray in your private room."

The way of the gods, in the old Shinto religion, is to entrust everything to the Cosmos cells. Muscle cells cannot produce muscles. There is no such thing as genes for muscle cells. Cosmos cells control cell metabolism. Scientists say that DNA is contained in the right brain. Actually, DNA does not exist within the body, but the memory of it resides within the mind. It is the memory of all lives and wisdoms of past reincarnations.

Jesus said that God is "closer than thy hands and feet." This means that the Cosmos cells, the cells that contain the complete genes of the almighty Creator, exist right behind our hearts.

Cells have the function of being both receiver and transmitter.

<Transmitting ill thoughts> Upon the transmission of ill thoughts, a quadruplet of them is received in turn. Sick cells grow rapidly, causing the body to lose control of those ill thoughts. This negative spiral emanates bad frequencies that are disliked by others.

<Transmission of nice thoughts> This leads to receiving more instructions and revelations from the heavenly world. Light (Aura) is emanated. More people are attracted to such a person.

Sick cells disappear and healthy cells increase. The body will receive cosmic energy and cosmic wisdom, glow with a brighter aura and have a halo. One's fate is decided in his or her mind. Whether the cells become healthy or sick depends on one's state of mind. This is the law of the universe. People say, God helps those who help themselves; his salvation is within himself.

Birds of a feather flock together

The astronauts who reached the moon had their bodies cleansed by the power of the moon's strong energy force and gained heightened intuition for greater inspiration, revelation and insight. It is good to be in the company of people who connect with the universe. If you can pray for the salvation of human beings, you should be able to solve any difficulties (even massive debts). Nothing is impossible with God.

Prayer and meditation connect us with the heavenly world. Without the mind to ask God for help, Satan would soon take over. Silently tell Satan to go away in the name of God.

When you strongly believe that you have been given the right to be treated and healed, you are given the mercy of God to remove illnesses and/or haunting spirits. You can even save others from Satan.

Jesus said, "Be gone, Satan! For it is written, 'You shall worship the Lord your God and him only shall you serve.'" It is important to fully understand the mystery of the human body.

3. On atoms, electrons and health
(1) The harm of pesticides

① Pesticide sprays contaminate air and soil equally. Contamination of air and soil lead to contamination of water. When nature is contaminated, the toxins spread over a large area, making it difficult to clean up.
Many would say that contaminated water will destroy humanity before nuclear weapons will. 75% of the human body is water, therefore the pollution of water becomes pollution of the body.

② Pesticides kill the microbes on leaves and fruits. The amino acids contained in plants are created by microbes. Fewer microbes in vegetables mean they have poorer nutritional value. Vitamins are essentially the living microbes, and they are lacking in those pesticide-laden vegetables. Since mineral components are also created by microbes, these vegetables contain fewer minerals as well.

③ Pesticides are acidic, turning naturally-alkaline vegetables acidic, which in turn spoils the blood when consumed. Acidic vegetables cause bloating and upset stomach. This is because pesticides spoil cells in the body and generate carbon dioxide gas. The acid contained in pesticides causes the body to become excessively acidic. The body tries to neutralize itself by forcibly releasing oxygen. Oxygen is life energy itself. The shortage of oxygen then causes illnesses such as cancer and atopic dermatitis. Spoilage of blood is known as "o-ketsu" (clotted blood) in Chinese medicine, and is considered to be the cause of numerous diseases.

④ Cabbages grow layers of leaves. They tend to contain the highest amount of pesticides of all vegetables. Green juice usually contains kale as one of the ingredients. Kale attracts insects. Which means the green juice made from pesticide-laden vegetables is the most dangerous juice of all.

⑤ Using pesticides for growing vegetables is the same as putting pesticides on humans. It is essentially an indirect murder. Humans cannot survive when the air, soil and water are contaminated. It is like leading us to a collective suicide. You will be charged with murder if you force a person to drink pesticide, yet nobody will criticize a farmer who sprays pesticides on his crop. I find it rather odd.

⑥ What helps plants grow are the microbes living in the leaves and the soil. Plant roots absorb nutrients from dead microbes in the soil. They are rich in protein and minerals. They are the organic matter. When the protein is carried up to the leaves, the aerobic bacteria living in the leaves turn it into amino acids. Carbon dioxide and methane gas are converted into oxygen. This is the mechanism of photosynthetic reaction. It is actually done by the aerobic bacteria, not chlorophyll.

⑦ Pesticides damage and kill the microbes in the leaves and soil. The roots cannot absorb nutrients, causing malnutrition. This is when pests attack and diseases break out. As the number of microbes in leaves decreases, photosynthetic capacity drops. Amino acids are not produced, preventing the plants from growing properly. In turn, the ability for nature to supply oxygen decreases. This is how the destruction of nature progresses.

⑧ Radiation is highly acidic. Dipping fruits and vegetables in strong alkaline water of pH 10 to 11 for 20 seconds will neutralize them. They will taste great, as they used to taste a long time ago, without bitterness. When you dip leafy vegetables such as spinach into alkaline water, the leaves will perk up and stay fresh longer.

(2) Going back to health

① Humans consist of mostly water. Water accounts for 75% to 80% of our body's mass. Water (H_2O) is made of oxygen and hydrogen, therefore we are mostly oxygen (acidic, positive pole) and hydrogen (alkaline, negative pole). Our lives are the fine balance of oxygen and hydrogen. We become sick if the balance is disrupted.

② When a patient is told by a doctor that he or she has one week to live, neutralizing 75% of his or her bodily fluid will cease the progress of the disease. The human body functions correctly in a neutral state. In a mother's womb, the fetus grows to its full size within nine months. When the mother's amniotic fluid is neutral, the fetus grows healthily. When the amniotic fluid spoils due to less oxygen, the fetus is affected. The baby will later develop symptoms like atopic dermatitis or allergies. When the amniotic fluid is lacking oxygen, supplementing it with oxygen and aerobic bacteria (containing oxygen) will return it to a neutral state.

③ All substances are formed from atoms and electrons, energy and mass. Oxygen and hydrogen fill the cosmic space and are in perfect balance. Oxygen is energy and hydrogen is mass. Oxygen is life energy itself. Hydrogen is the body itself. Human beings consist of life, spiritual energy and the body. Oxygen is not a substance with mass; it always exists as gas and light.

④ Human beings stay alive by breathing in oxygen. Since oxygen is life energy itself, it is important when practicing Prāṇāyāma to be mindful that you are inhaling the life energy within the air, and not merely breathing unconsciously. This way, your body will be supplemented with oxygen, which is life energy itself.

⑤ The atmosphere is intangible and holistic. It is the almighty life energy. There is only one source of energy: the infinite energy of the universe. The universe is this single, infinite energy. People tend to believe that they each have their own, unique life energy. This way of thinking is burdensome. Modern people are deluded to think that their physical body is the only life form. They overlook what gives them their life. They believe that their physical body, which contains no energy to begin with, is what they are. This leads to illnesses. Illness is the shortage of energy. Disease comes from minds, as well as the lack of energy.

⑥ There is only one source of life: consciousness and energy in the universe. The Creator creates everything, and dwells in all as energy and mass. The Creator is almighty and immortal. His every creation is nothing short of perfection. A human's life is the alter ego, spirit and soul of the Creator. A human's life is linked with that of the Creator. Severing this line of connection means instant death.

⑦ When I speak of oxygen, I refer to the oxygen of aerobic bacteria. Hydrogen, in the same sense, is of anaerobic bacteria. The balance of the physical condition of the body is also the balance of microbes within. To lose the balance between aerobic bacteria and anaerobic bacteria is to break the balance between oxygen and hydrogen. This is the cause of diseases. Aerobic bacteria convert carbon dioxide and methane gas within the body into the life energy of oxygen by photosynthesis. Oxygen deficiency degrades tissue and blood, causing cancer, atopic dermatitis or various intractable diseases.

If you break the law of the harmony of the universe, or the law of love, you become ill.

⑧ Countless microbes inhabit the air, water and soil. Approximately 8,000 trillion microbes live in a human body; their assembly is the human body. Red and white blood cells, as well as lymphocytes, are also microbes. Soil fertilizer comes through the food we eat, feeding the myriad of microbes. Since modern people ignore the work of microbes, they mindlessly destroy nature and their own health. Not understanding the existence and effects of microbes is the black spot on the natural sciences.

⑨ It is microbes that create, maintain, and manage nature, and decompose and treat waste. This earth and mankind cannot exist without the microbes being in balance.
Modern science does not know of the fact that the combination of aerobic and anaerobic bacteria in the body create blood, muscle and bones in about 3 minutes at ambient temperature.

⑩ Cooking vegetables and organic foods at high heat or in a microwave oven turns them into food with dead microbes. The health benefits of these vegetables and other foods are lost. Fresh vegetables are oxygen-rich. What is important is not the number of calories, but the amount or lack of energy or oxygen. Oxygen-deficient vegetables and foods spoil quickly. The common sense of the modern human being is all wrong.

(3) Earth's rotation and health

① The balance between oxygen and hydrogen is achieved
through the two rotational movements of light energy.
Energy is always generated in a whirl. As a result, the light
element of oxygen works to combine atoms and electrons to
create objects. This rotational motion is called an ionization
reaction, or ion exchange.

+Oxygen ⟳ Emission, release ---- dispersion, collapse

−Hydrogen ⟲ Aspiration, pulling ---- bonding, composition

The difference in the rotational direction simply depends
at which angle you look at it. Viewing it as one will reveal
the repeating pull and release action, releasing the electric
energy.

② The ion exchange of oxygen and hydrogen generates heat by
the rotation of a light emitting pulse, which in turn heats up
by means of the friction of cells. The normal body temperature is kept at around 36.5 ℃. The higher the electric energy
is, and the better balanced the positive and negative charges,
the faster the 'motor' runs, keeping a better circulation
within the body. This state contributes to faster metabolism,
more efficient delivery of oxygen and nutrients and better
removal of waste within the body.

③ Lower electric energy means a slower 'motor', poorer circulation and eventually, sickness. When the electrical state in the blood worsens, waste (cholesterol) tends to build up. It clogs veins, causing high blood pressure. Clogged blood vessels prevent blood to pass through, and sometimes rupture. In the intestines, escherichia coli cleans the interior, but when the electrical condition worsens, the bacteria become sluggish, causing constipation or fecal impaction.

④ Energy is always generated in a whirl.
High pressure is dextral ---- releasing, active.
Low pressure is sinistral --- pulling.
The earth's energy is pulled away from the body and lost.
Asthma and susceptibility to illness occur due to lack of energy.
A person is born at high pressure and dies at low pressure.

Sinistral --- pull   Dextral --- release, giving

⑤ Within the human body, the right side is positive, and the left, negative. The upper body is positive and the lower body is negative. It is a cross.
Right hand is positive, the north pole and releasing; left hand is negative, south pole and pulling. Ksitigarbha statues usually hold the right hand up and left hand flat. There is an ion exchange going on by releasing energy from the right hand and pulling it in from the left. So, when passing objects to people, always use your right hand, which represents releasing, and receive with left, for pulling in.
In any culture in the world, prayer is done by putting both

hands together. The center between positive and negative is neutral. We all know unconsciously that nature and God are neutral.

⑥ When oxygen and hydrogen are balanced, they are at a state of ± 0, or neutrality. This is how a neutron is. Permanent energy is generated from the molecules of light in that state. The word Namu (南無), as part of the Buddhists' prayers, ultimately hints at the balanced state of oxygen and hydrogen. Neutrons create all things. Elemental transmutation means that one atom and more than one electron are bound together.

⑦ The active agents in elemental transmutation at normal temperature are the microbes. Since microbes have telepathic abilities, they can read human consciousness. The laws of microbes are cooperation, sharing and no-conflict. Unless you are a conscious person you cannot get the benefit of the microbe. For those with high consciousness, microbes work very well. People tend to clash. By imitating those in conflict, cells begin eating the adjacent cells and start growing larger. They turn into cancer cells.

⑧ Understanding and applying the principle of elemental transmutation at room temperature makes it possible to be creative. Using the power of creation during recession is the way to survive in those hard times. There is an infinite supply of atoms and electrons. There is no shortage of materials; they are low cost and safe. No recession in that regard. The rotational movement of the light circles is infinite.

People tend to think that energy is finite. Energy is, as a matter of fact, infinite and eternal. People do not understand this yet.

⑨ In the natural world things are created through the perfect balance of oxygen (Yang) and hydrogen (Yin). $1 + 1 = 1 \pm 0$. Neutral

This is fusion or binding. Objects are created by a fusion or binding reaction. However, the chemical substances that human beings create are made by dividing the molecular structure of those substances. They are made by decomposition and separation. This is different from the fusion reaction; therefore chemical substances always have side-effects. Separated things are then mushed into one substance. These single substances are different from what was created by fusion, and they always have side-effects.

⑩ Humans are made of life and the physical body. But modern people think that the physical body IS the person himself. When the mind is shifted to the negative state it causes discordance. And, because it generates less energy, these people are susceptible to illnesses.

The more discordant the world is, the more diseases spread through the world. Doctors have no idea of the true cause of diseases. They try to deal with diseases with symptomatic therapy. But because the cause is not eliminated, more illnesses occur one after another.

(4) The arrival of the era of curing intractable diseases by ourselves

Messages from the heavenly world

In the previous chapters I mentioned that the Earth has entered a stronger energy area.

There is a purpose for this move. When the energy gets stronger, humans will be divided into lower-energy people and higher-energy people. It is like parting the curtains. This is what has been described as ascension and the photon belt.

People with high sensibility are the ones with higher energy. As this type of people's energy becomes stronger, their sensibility will also become more heightened, turning them into even more cognizant, rational people.

People with low sensibility are the ones with low energy. They are the sickly type, who cannot tolerate high energy and become sicker and sicker; their minds snap, and they might commit crimes, alienate others, become confrontational or cause harm to others. This is the emotional-type. A highly sensitive person is willing to help others in need.

It is December 2016 as I write this. The energy of the Earth will further increase in 2017. The energy is trying to promote human evolution. The heavenly world has programmed the evolution of mankind from the emotional type to the rational type. Emotional-type people are selfish, always confrontational and trying to alienate others. They are the type to insist on a money-, material- and self-centered lifestyle.

They are the very ones who elected President Trump, or who ousted Moderati in Italy.

The Utopian society is coming soon. It is a society of coexistence, mutual respect and sharing. In this society, those who are disturbing others or not needed will be eliminated. The 26,000-year cycle of astrological ages is about to come around to Judgement Day. The lost continents of Mu, Atlantis and Lemuria all disappeared at this particular moment in the astrological age cycle. It is simply a historical fact. Now is the time for Judgment Day. Higher consciousness equals higher energy. A community of only highly conscious people will become the Utopian society of coexistence, mutual respect and sharing.

A person with high energy understands that he receives the benefit of infinite cosmic life. Whoever recognizes the existence of this infinite cosmic life and incorporates it into the body can pass the final judgment. There are publications on the teachings of White Eagle. The cause of any illness is the deficit of spiritual light in the body. Disease is the stress of the mind manifesting as physical stress.

People have illusions that the physical body is alive, and that the body is themselves. They forget that life controls the body. Disharmony between life and body, imbalance between hormones and the body, are the cause of various illnesses. A poor mind is the reflection of a lower consciousness; it is deficient in light energy.

All diseases can be treated by light therapy. There are cosmic rays that can cure diseases. When light energy is readily accepted, the seven chakras of the human body are activated, and diseases can be treated with the ultimate light energy and the wave lengths of light.

When a sick person connects the center of love with the energy of light, he is instantly cured. This is because the person unconsciously is able to select the white light and the wave length that his/her soul and body need.

Without this white light therapy device, the human race will be extinct. This device is offered by the Global Family. When our White Light Generator is installed at home, any illness will disappear within six weeks. The mind is released from the body. Anyone with this device will be able to think positively and start seeking brighter things, therefore their lives will be much brighter. Negative thoughts will disappear. Then, they will attract only good things.

On this Earth there live people with all kinds of different ideas. There are dark, crude wavelengths that seek darkness, and exquisite wavelengths seeking light. Thousands of people emit thousands of different wavelengths. It is only a matter of which wavelength the person him/herself wishes to tune in to.

If you seek darkness, you will be surrounded by darkness. It will attract protests, disasters and accidents. When seeking light, light will be given. It's your choice.

The heavenly world demands the evolution of mankind from the emotional type to the rational type. The outdated emotional type of people are in conflict with others. These self-centered people get in the way of the establishment of the Utopian society. Therefore they are regarded as unnecessary and will be eliminated.

In order to help mankind evolve to the rational stage as a whole, since whoever is ill with low energy cannot catch up, they will be eliminated. For that reason, the heavenly world always sends messages and useful information to help us heal even the intractable diseases.

Even better, there are ways to heal ourselves, without depending on medical institutions. I mentioned various causes of illnesses. The cause of dementia, intractable diseases and stroke is contaminated blood. It is necessary to improve blood circulation in the brain and to clear up the thickened blood and the contaminants within cancer cells.

In a humidifier tank, mix two parts water to one part fermented broth made with medicinal herbs, and inhale the steam. Inhaling it through your nose will immediately improve blood circulation in the brain. Dementia should be improved.

If you inhale the steam through your mouth, it will immediately flow to the lungs and will be absorbed by the blood vessels concentrated in them. Within a few hours, oxygen circulates through the whole body, neutralizing and thinning the blood. Furthermore, since aerobic bacteria that carry oxygen, capable of creating blood, tissue and bones within three minutes, will improve the blood throughout the body, any decay is reversed on the spot. Even things like cancer symptoms will immediately be neutralized so that the person will regain his/her health right away.

Wavelengths of 8,000 to 10,000 hertz neutralize thickened and contaminated blood and tumors. Blood thins to a normal level. Tumors will be dissolved. Aerobic bacteria in contact with the leaves of medicinal herbs have medicinal components. They combine with anaerobic bacteria inside the body to create blood, tissue and bones within three minutes at ambient temperature. Since the combination of aerobic and anaerobic bacteria neutralize all toxic substances within the body, various medical conditions begin to heal.

Because the cause of the disease is gone, people will be free of diseases. The microbes living on the leaves of herbs make saponins and other useful medicinal ingredients, such as amino acids and minerals.

When microbes living in the leaves of cordyceps sinensis or

ginseng are transferred to spinach, you can grow spinach with added medicinal components. It is, indeed, medicine and food in one.

Epilogue

The universe and the natural world are under the law of the absolute truth and its quintessence. This law is reproducible without fail. The heavenly world, the world of God and the Shambhala council control the entirety of God's will, His program and the adherence to the law of the universe. This law of the universe is what we call God.

However, most people are unaware of this law, thus fail to live in conformity to the law. When such discord happens, they utter, "Oh my God!"

I am happy that I am able to present to you the very first book in the world to describe the wisdom of the realm of God. I would like to express my sincere gratitude to all of whom helped me publish this book.

May God bless you!

Masaru Kawai

www.ingramcontent.com/pod-product-compliance
Lightning Source LLC
Chambersburg PA
CBHW032003080426
42735CB00007B/499